STOP DROP ROLL and SMILE

for Migraine Relief

How to Stop Headache and Migraine Pain Without Drugs

DIANA ANDERSON

Stop, Drop, Roll, and Smile for Migraine Relief
How to Stop Headache and Migraine Pain Without Drugs
Diana Anderson © 2019

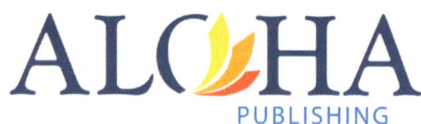

Print ISBN: 978-1-61206-191-7
PDF eBook ISBN: 978-1-61206-192-4

Interior and Cover Design by: Fusion Creative Works, FusionCW.com
Lead Editor: Jennifer Regner

For more information, visit RealMigraineSolutions.com

To purchase this book at discounted prices, go to AlohaPublishing.com

Published by

ALOHA
PUBLISHING

Printed in the United States of America

CONTENTS

Regardless of the underlying cause of your headache or migraine, be it a hangover, a food or weather trigger, stress, or some other issue, head pain always comes from the same source problem: the nervous system is overtaxed and has run out of the critical resources it needs to function—and/or it needs to rest to renew the cells in the nervous system.

If you have sought help from other resources without success, you will find what you need here. This short, simple guide is unique, and it will give you much-needed answers with specific directions to help you relieve your pain quickly. Give it a try.

Many others have used these simple steps with excellent results. I hope this material helps you as well.

I FOUND WAYS TO STOP A MIGRAINE HEADACHE WITHOUT DRUGS—AND THEY WORK FOR OTHER HEADACHES TOO.

HOW TO STOP A HEADACHE

Everyone has headaches—"regular" headaches or migraines. Twelve percent of the population worldwide suffers from migraines, and migraines are a leading cause of absences from work in the U.S.[1]

Any headache disrupts your day and makes it harder for you to function and perform. Migraines disrupt your *life*. If you or someone you love has migraines or frequent head pain, nothing is more important than relieving or preventing that suffering.

After 30 years of suffering from migraines, I was experiencing them on an almost daily basis. I had to find a way to heal myself—because the prescriptions weren't working. I was desperate to get my life back.

It took me over two years, but I finally healed myself from migraine pain. The first step was stopping the prescriptions. Along the way, I found ways to stop a migraine in its tracks without any drugs. And I learned that my methods work for "regular" headaches too. Many friends, family members, and students have benefited from my methods.

Most importantly, I learned that a migraine headache is an emergency message from your brain, signaling that you are lacking critical resources your brain needs.

STOP: YOU ARE GETTING A MIGRAINE BECAUSE YOUR BRAIN IS OVERTAXED, UNDERNOURISHED, AND IT NEEDS REST.

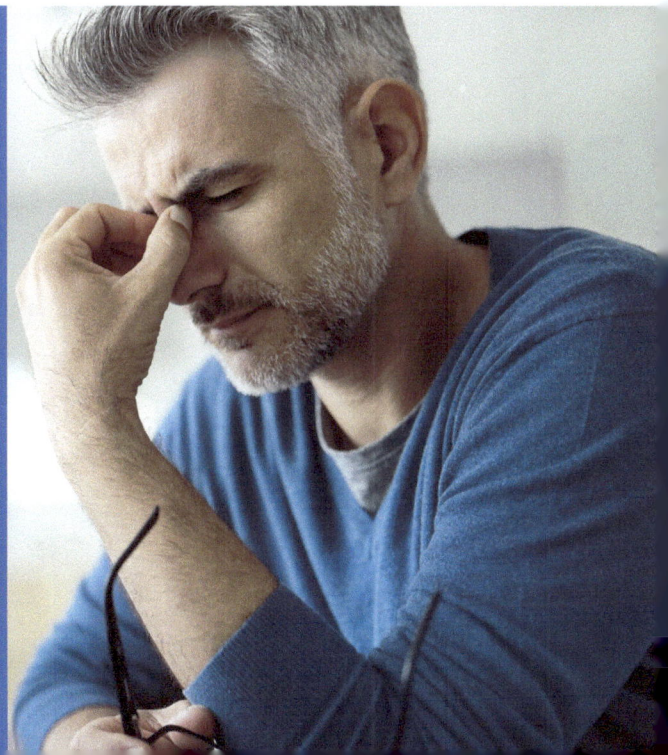

STOP, DROP, ROLL, AND SMILE

You don't need a prescription to cover up the pain; you must simply give your nervous system what it needs. This manual shows you how to prevent a developing headache from reaching its painful potential.

The concept of "Stop, Drop, and Roll" has been used for generations by the National Fire Prevention Agency (NFPA) to teach children what to do if their clothes catch on fire. They need to follow these simple steps:

1.   STOP, don't run.

2.   DROP to the ground.

3.   ROLL on the ground to smother the flames.

Millions of people remember these words. I borrowed the phrase to make it easy to remember, by comparing a migraine to a fire. Even if you've never heard of this technique, hopefully the words will be etched in your mind by the end of this manual.

A migraine is similar to a fire. It starts small and can quickly get out of control. When a flame is small, extinguishing it is easy. As with any blaze, once it is a raging, forest-fire-sized migraine, it takes a lot more time and resources to put out those hot flames.

Begin at the first signs to stop the fire from spreading and you will conquer it. Otherwise, it might have to burn itself out over a few days.

For immediate relief from a migraine, here is a quick formula that works when a migraine is just beginning. This method addresses the underlying causes of headaches including hydration, nutrients, health issues, and physical and emotional stress.

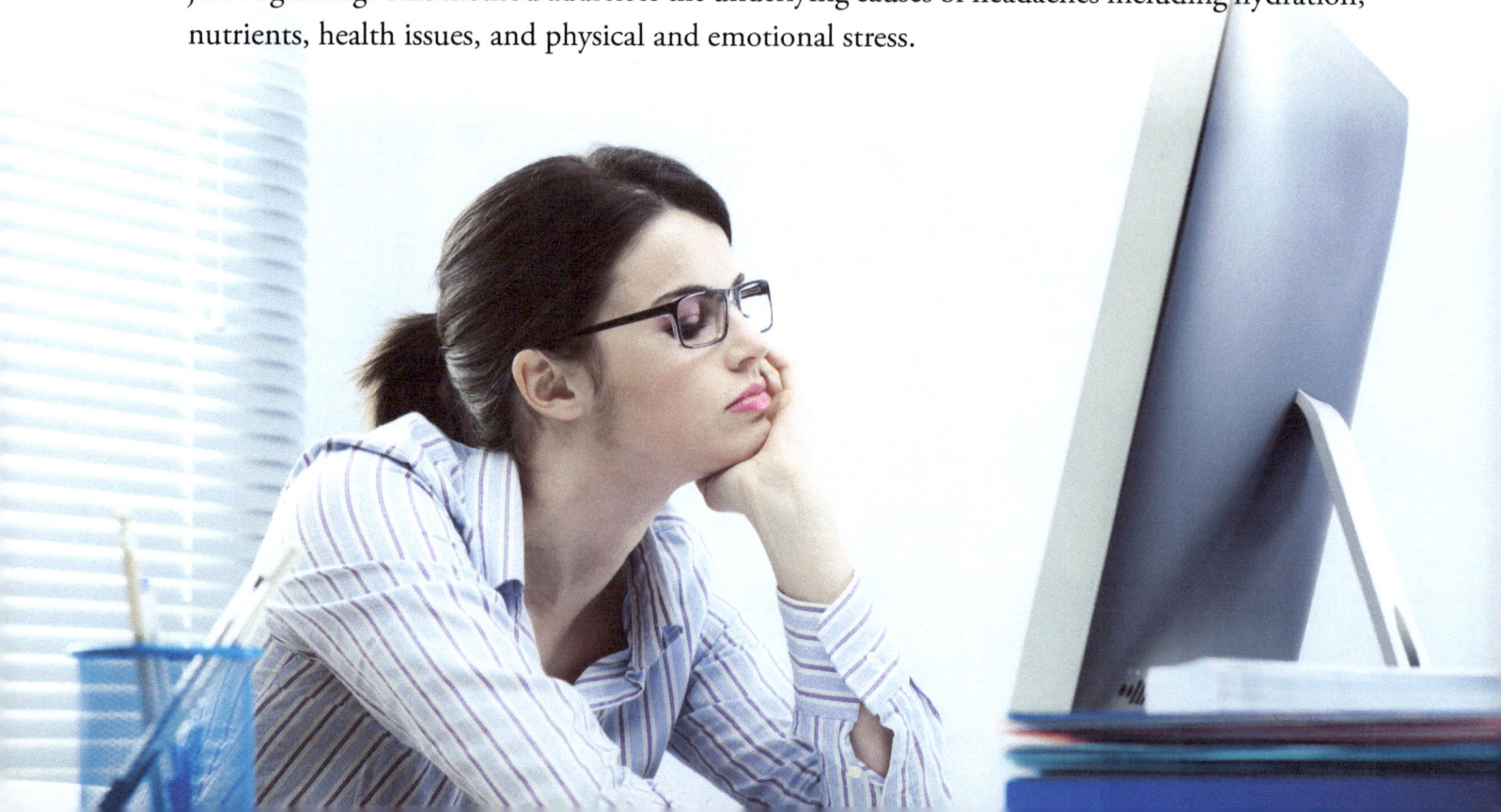

STOP
DROP
ROLL
SMILE

1. **STOP** what you are doing so you can be completely present with your current physical state and stop stimulating the nervous system. No phone, no computer, no TV. Provide super hydration that your brain and body need, right now. ("Super" hydration is water with natural glucose and minerals from juices or high water-content fruits such as orange juice, coconut water, celery or celery juice, or watermelon. See the Bonus Material for more details.)

2. **DROP** your breath into your belly and breathe as you expand your diaphragm with slow, calm, deep breaths. Drop your awareness into your body.

3. **ROLL** out the tension in your shoulders on a foam roller or hard surface edge, or get someone to give you 10 minutes of deep shoulder, neck, and back rubbing. You can also do any of the listed relaxation techniques (see ROLL section). Relax the jaw, drop the shoulders, and focus on calming your emotions. Move the spine to circulate the spinal fluid.

4. **SMILE** and feel gratitude to wash away cortisol. The act of smiling and feeling gratitude releases serotonin, which replaces the stress hormone cortisol. Think of things and people in your life you are thankful for.

This is so important I am saying it again: *Understand that a migraine is a cry for help from your body.* You can relieve a headache by "fixing" or satisfying the underlying causes. A significant part of this is relaxing your body to shift it into a calm state. When you provide your body what it needs, the headaches will be greatly diminished and can go away completely.

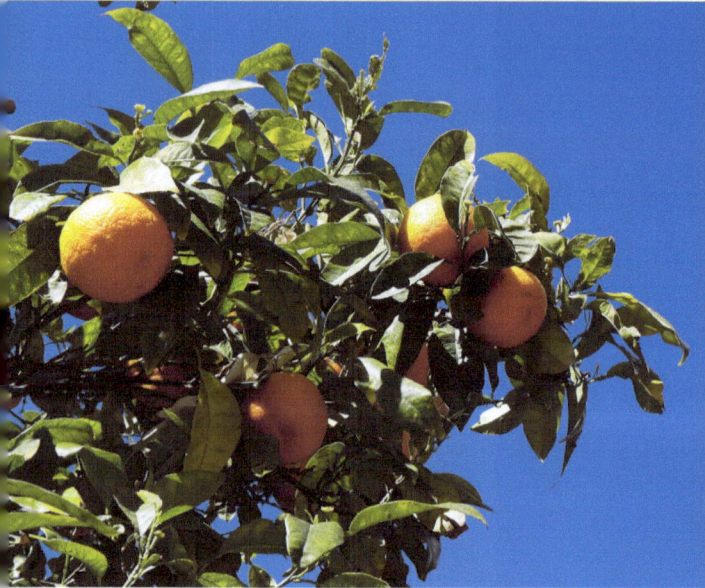

STOP, DROP, ROLL, AND SMILE WILL HELP RELAX YOUR BODY AND MOVE YOU OUT OF A STRESSED FIGHT-OR-FLIGHT MODE.

Tension and stress contribute to the developing headache. You may also need to hydrate your body and provide it with nutrients—glucose and minerals, specifically. As a preventative measure, simply staying more hydrated with water also helps.

The next chapters explain more about the causes of headaches and how to use this method most effectively.

STOP
DROP
ROLL
SMILE

WHY HEAD PAIN?

Your brain uses a tremendous amount of the resources you take in. Although it weighs only about 3 pounds, it uses 20 percent of your oxygen[2] and hydration, and as much as 60 to 70 percent of your glucose.[3] The more active your brain is, the more fuel it needs. When you are working at the computer, doing creative tasks for hours, thinking hard, engaged in conversation, or talking to a group of people, your brain needs large amounts of oxygen and nutrients.

The more stimulation to your nervous systems, such as sounds, lights, computers, people, thinking tasks, et cetera, the more your brain will use up resources.

THE SIMPLISTIC EXPLANATION OF WHAT CAUSES MIGRAINES IS A LACK OF RESOURCES TO THE BRAIN.

STRESS DEMANDS EVEN MORE RESOURCES AND CAN REDIRECT THOSE RESOURCES AWAY FROM THE BRAIN.

Stress of any kind causes the brain and body to use resources even more quickly. Like a race car, it must refuel often or it will run out of gas.

You may be under stress without consciously realizing it. Sometimes stress can activate your body's fight-or-flight response (through your *sympathetic* nervous system), and this is the most common cause for depletion of resources to the brain. Your body will divert resources from your brain to your muscles. If your nervous system is in fight-or-flight mode for an extended period, your brain can run out of fuel and won't be able to function.

A MIGRAINE IS THE BRAIN SENDING A DISTRESS CALL TO THE BODY TO SEND MORE RESOURCES FAST. THE RESULT IS PAIN, CAUSED BY AN OVERSTIMULATED NERVOUS SYSTEM AND A LACK OF RESOURCES: *OXYGEN, MINERALS, HYDRATION, GLUCOSE, AND SPINAL FLUID FLOW.*

12

The central nervous system and your brain depend on these nutrients to function. When you are low on any of them, it is like operating the nervous system on fumes, with the nerves literally starving.

Pain medications simply block the symptoms of your headache. Once you understand that migraines are an indicator that your brain is running on fumes, you also understand that pain medications do not address any of the issues—and in fact, they can make your headaches worse or more frequent.

The real solution is to rest the nervous system and replenish the supplies (oxygen, minerals, glucose, and hydration). **Stop, Drop, Roll, and Smile is a way to relax and refuel.**

So many people who get headaches or migraines are not resupplying the nervous system when it asks for it. Additionally, if the liver, neck, blood, or blood vessels have underlying issues (I will describe these later), then less of the available resources might make it to the brain.

Fight-or-flight mode can be caused by stress, tension, and any issue in the body that the nervous system interprets as a threat. A critical concept to understand is that **all migraines occur when your body is in fight-or-flight mode.** If your body is in fight-or-flight mode for too long or too often, resources are consumed faster.

If you have migraine headaches often, your body is dealing with other issues that make your symptoms worse, and further changes are needed to heal the body and stop getting migraines for good. For long-term healing, see "Commit to the Cure" for more on how you can start this journey.

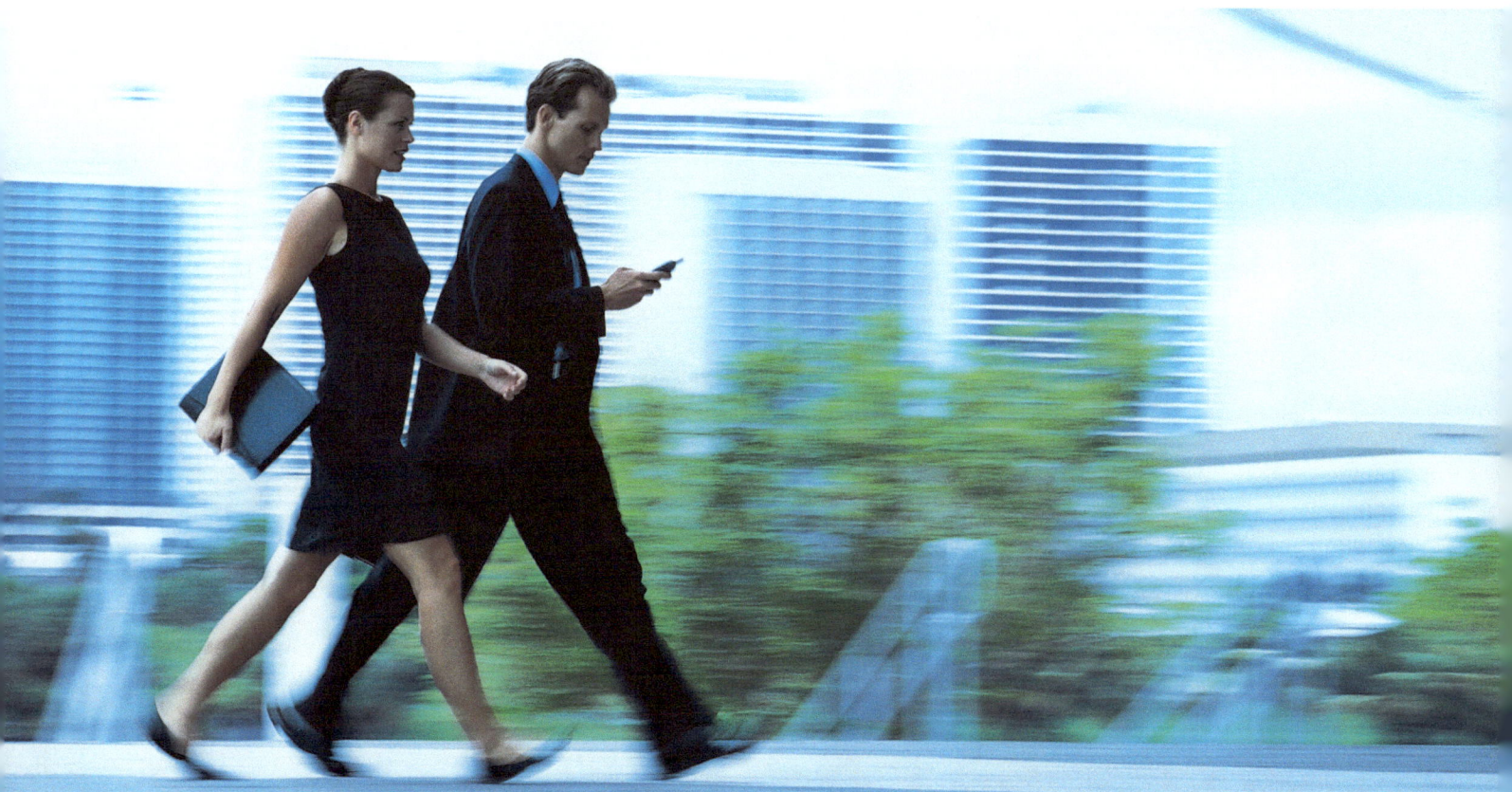

HOW IT STARTS

Have you ever noticed while sitting at a computer to do a major task that suddenly you can't focus? Lack of focus can come from a lack of fuel to the brain, which is glucose. Eating some fruit would be an excellent, healthy choice for most people.

If you are sitting at your desk and you feel very tired in the middle of the day, with or without focus problems, the most likely reason is lack of oxygen to the brain and other tissues in the body. The best thing you can do is stand up, wiggle, twist, raise your arms up and down, and breathe deeply. If possible, jog in place or go for a walk and increase your oxygen intake. *Qigong* is the most effect exercise to increase oxygen flow. Undulating your spine is also very helpful. This increases blood flow to your back muscles and improves flow of both blood and spinal fluid to your brain (for more information about Qigong, see https://www.nqa.org/what-is-qigong-).

These things can help you any time and may head off a migraine before you even need to *Stop, Drop, Roll and Smile.*

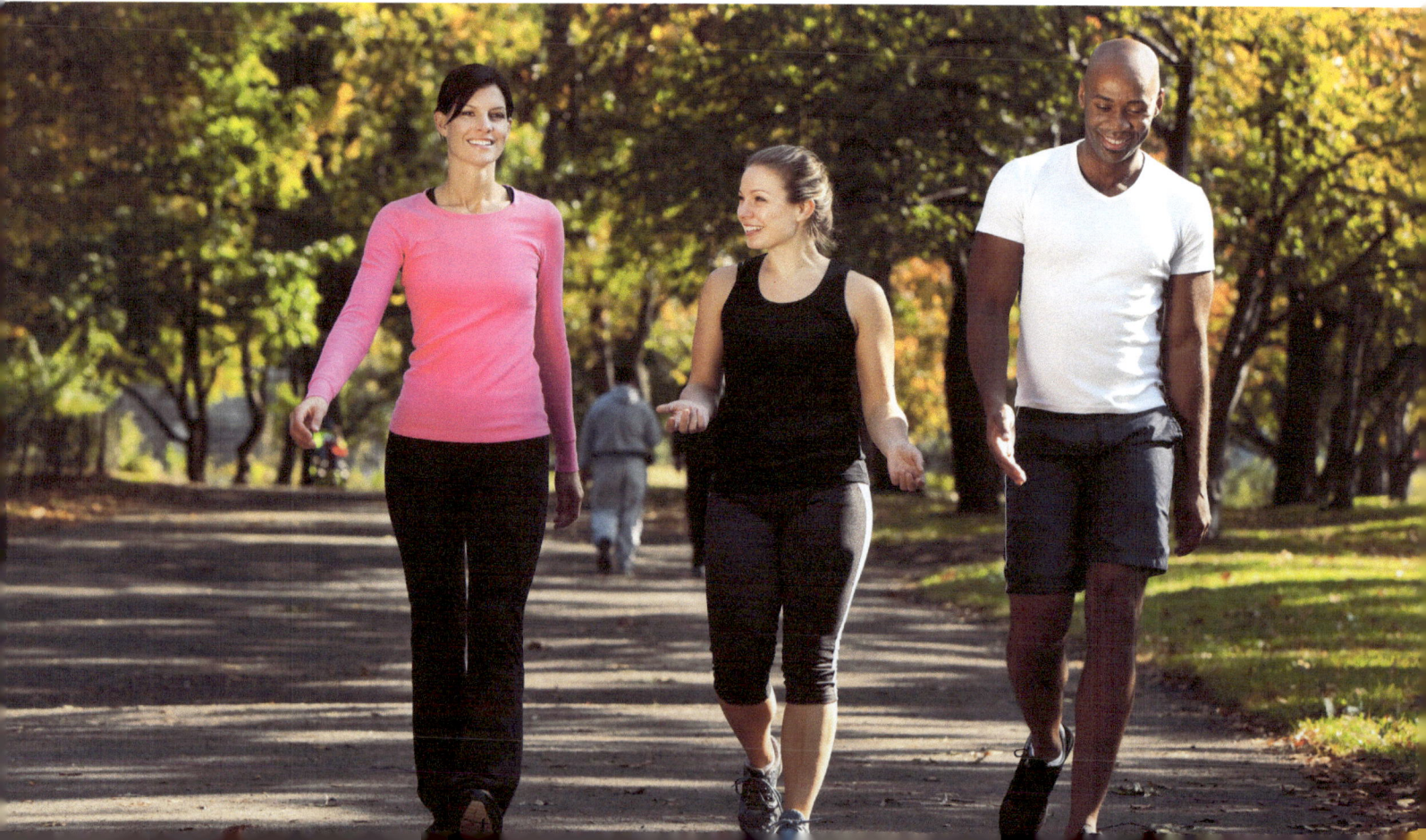

WARNING SIGNS OF A DEVELOPING MIGRAINE

Regardless of what caused your nervous system to be overstimulated and under-supplied, you need to be able to recognize when a migraine is beginning.

You may already know what your warning signs are. But if you don't, here are some possible indicators that a migraine could be coming your way:

- Lack of focus (due to low glucose, and the liver isn't working on sending more)

- Yawning (due to low oxygen levels reaching the brain)

- Eye or sinus pain developing without signs of infection (due to pinched nerve or blood vessels)

- Tight chest muscles, so that you are unable to take a deep breath (due to stress, tension, shallow breathing, and not exhaling carbon dioxide)

- Pain at the base of the skull (due to tight jaw)

- Neck and shoulder pain (due to shallow breathing or stress)

- Vision issues, nausea, weakness, or fatigue (because your nervous system is stuck in fight-or-flight mode)

- Feeling anxious (due to overstimulation of the nervous system, shallow breathing, and fight or flight)

- Tightness all over the body (due to dehydration and low oxygen combination)

- Increased heart rate (a sign you are in a sympathetic state/fight or flight)

- Shallow breathing

- Jaw tension or pain and/or ear pain or tightness

- Feeling pressure inside your head or "hot in the head"

- Loss of appetite

If you have any of these potential signs or your own early migraine symptoms, ***please Stop, Drop, Roll,*** and ***Smile***.

HOW TO RECOGNIZE FIGHT-OR-FLIGHT MODE

Have you ever noticed that when you are stressed, it is difficult to focus and think straight? This is because less oxygen and resources are flowing to the brain. In fight-or-flight mode, resources are directed to the muscles, lungs, and heart.

In the stressed mode of fight or flight, your body cannot rest and rejuvenate. You may be living in this state of hyperalertness without knowing it is happening—it can become a familiar pattern and your "normal." It is a state of chronic stress or pressure that has many health consequences. If this state of constant stress is combined with some of the other factors described later, especially with vascular issues, head trauma, or neck issues, then migraines can result.

If you are existing this way, you may think you can relax, but you are not reaching a full state of deep relaxation. This full relaxation is the state the body needs to reach to heal and recover. Living in a chronic state of stress taxes the body and prevents healing.

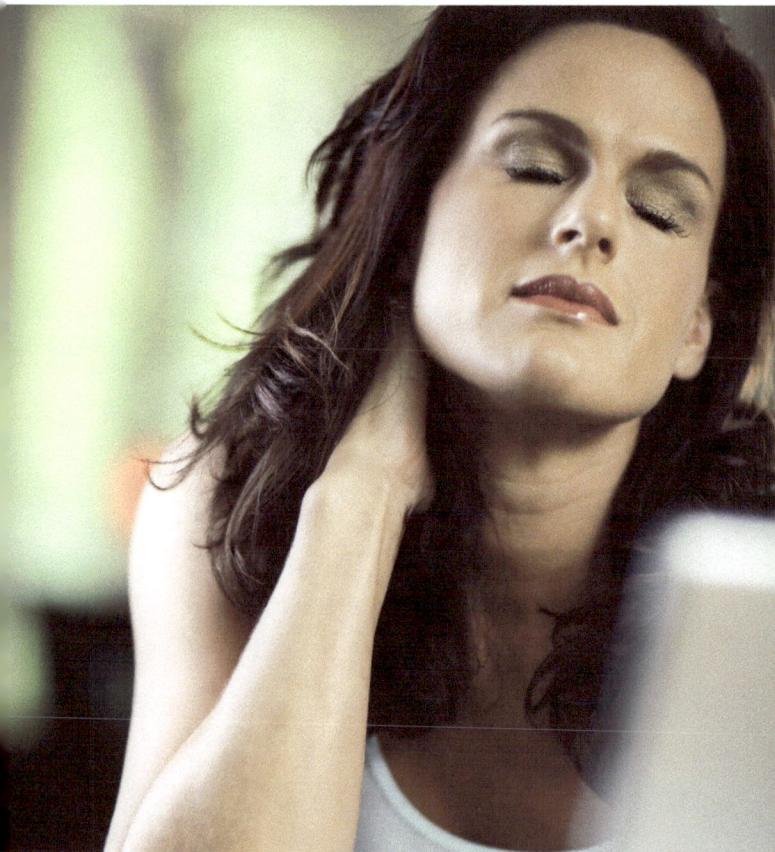

IF YOU EXPERIENCE FREQUENT HEADACHES OR MIGRAINES, YOU ARE NOT GETTING ENOUGH DEEP RELAXATION AND DOWNTIME FOR THE BODY AND NERVOUS SYSTEM TO HEAL AND RECOVER.

Other health issues are also an indication that this is happening. Later in the book, you will learn how to determine when you are fully relaxed and ways to help your body find a healthy "new normal" mode of operation.

WHAT HAPPENS IN FIGHT-OR-FLIGHT MODE

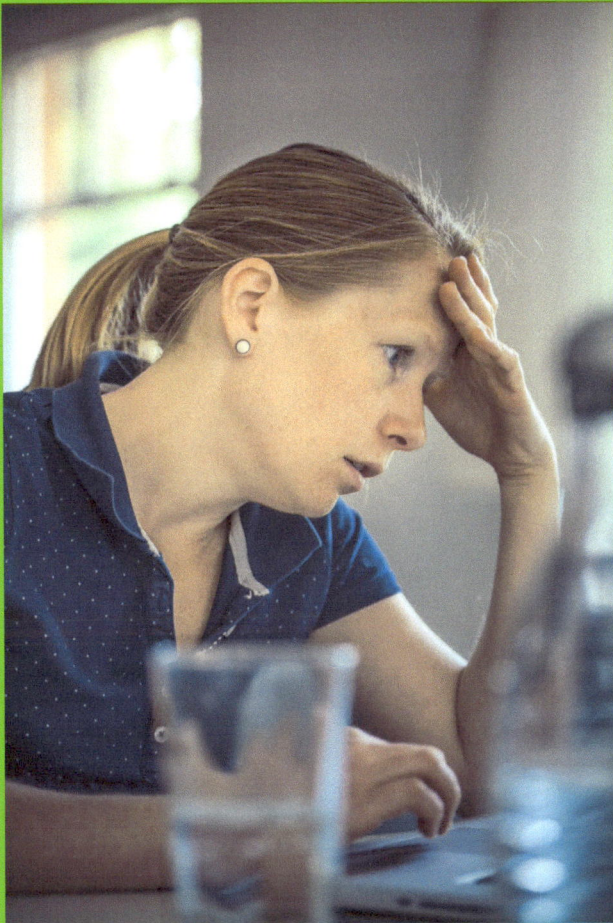

In fight-or-flight mode, your body takes quick, shallow breaths that increase the flow of blood to the body to provide ample oxygen to the muscles, in the event that your body must fight or flee to stay safe. Shallow breathing brings air into the upper half of the lungs. It keeps the body on guard and is known as the *sympathetic nervous system* mode.

You don't want to breathe this way all of the time for many reasons. It causes cortisol, a stress hormone, to be released into the body. Long term, this will damage your health. It also does not allow enough oxygen to your brain—it is meant to be temporary. Additionally, your body cannot grow new cells in this state. If you stay in this state for long periods of time, your cells are literally dying, with no cell replacement. In order to repair and rejuvenate your body, you need to be in "rest-and-digest" mode.

UNDERSTAND WHY *STOP, DROP, ROLL, AND SMILE* WORKS SO YOU CAN STOP THE MIGRAINE OR HEADACHE FROM DEVELOPING.

IN DEPTH:
STOP, DROP, ROLL, AND SMILE

What follows is more explanation of the four steps to stop a migraine or headache as it begins so you understand what is happening and can help your body. If done correctly, these four steps will mitigate a headache or migraine. If you experience frequent headaches, understand that you can heal your body and make migraines a problem of your past. See the Resources section for more information.

STOP

DROP

ROLL

SMILE

STOP WHAT YOU ARE DOING TO
SLOW DOWN THE STIMULATION
TO YOUR NERVOUS SYSTEM.

STEP 1:
STOP

If you recognize the signs of a migraine, your nervous system is overstimulated and lacks the resources it needs to function. You must immediately stop what you are doing to slow down the stimulation to your senses and nervous system.

WHAT TO DO RIGHT NOW

1. Stop working with electronics. Electronic screens are very stimulating to the nervous system and will require your brain to use more resources that you don't have available right now, so stop using phones, computers, TVs, and anything else with a monitor. Close your eyes and focus on relaxing your body and breathing.

Electronics give the wrong kind of stimulation and are the exact opposite of what you need to stop a migraine. **No electronics** until the threat is completely gone.

2. Stop to hydrate. When a migraine begins, you need to stop everything you are doing, stop stimulating the nervous system, and hydrate, hydrate, hydrate. This is regardless of what kind of migraine you have or of your underlying issues. You may not realize you are dehydrated, but a migraine happens because the brain is low on resources, and hydration is one of two ways those resources are carried to the brain.

For super hydration, drink liquids from nature:

- Plain, pure coconut water, with no sugar or preservatives added.
- Fresh fruit juice or fruits.
- Watermelon, or seasonal fruits and vegetables with a high water content.
- Celery has very high mineral and water content. It is excellent to eat on its own or you can make or buy celery juice for extra benefit.

Liquids that contain minerals can penetrate your cells so the glucose, nutrients, and hydration make it into the cells where they are needed. If you are lacking minerals, water alone won't be enough. I use the term "super" hydration to mean water with minerals and glucose.

Another option is to keep some small packets or a container of Emergen-C on hand. This is a powdered product that will give you minerals and glucose in a pinch when you can't get natural fruits and vegetables. If you are managing your blood sugar, in general stick to water and whole fruits and vegetables to avoid blood sugar spikes.

3. Step back from your immediate tasks and look inward. When a migraine is starting, you must shift the nervous system from fight or flight into a state of rest and digest, in order to stop the migraine from growing. Practice deep breathing and other forms of relaxation (more on this in Chapter Two).

All migraines happen in fight-or-flight mode. They cannot happen when you are in rest-and-digest mode (also called grow and renew because this is the state where you generate new cells). The first step to shifting into rest and digest is to stop what you are doing and become *present* with your body. Over time, you can easily learn how to monitor which state your nervous system is in and change it at will.

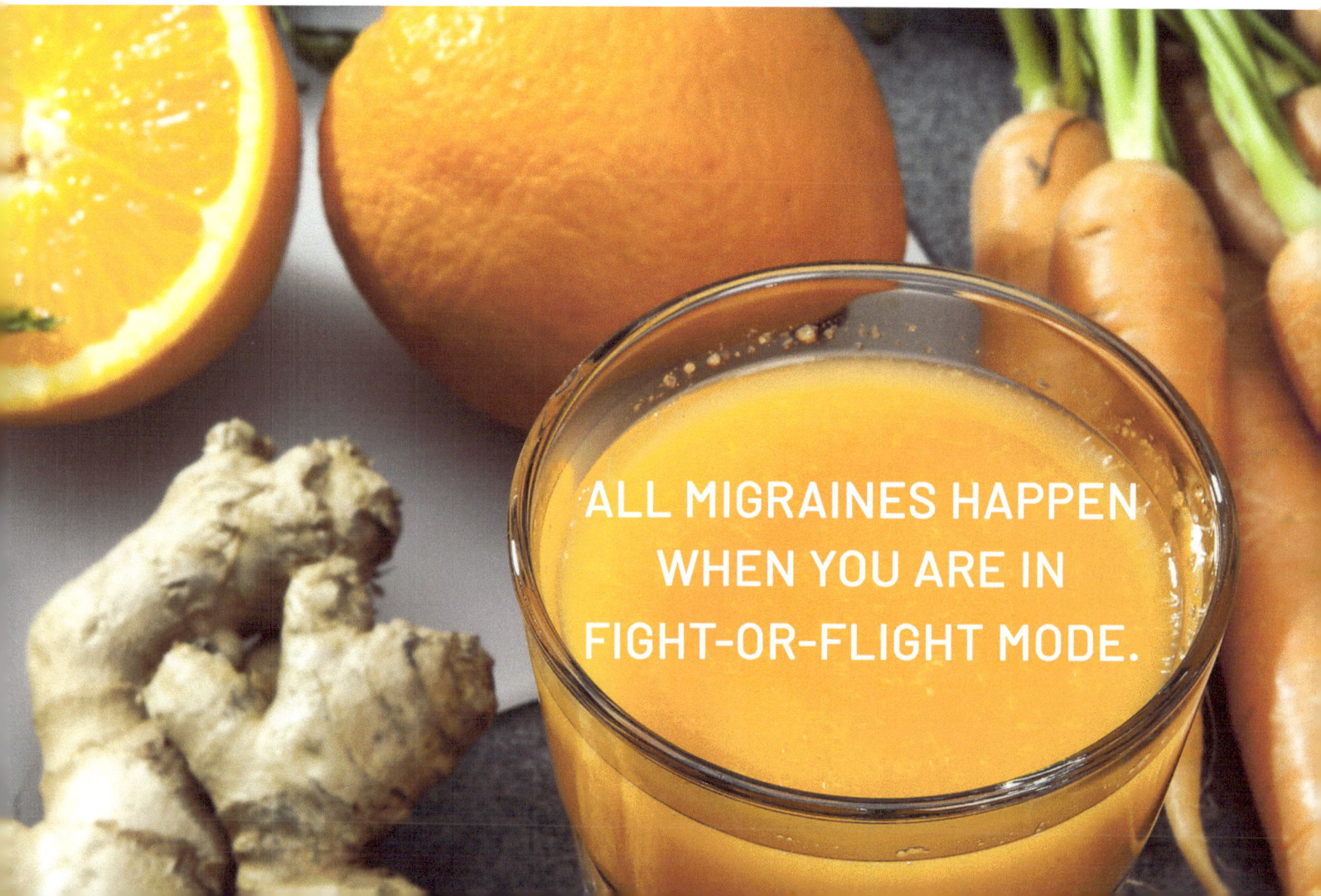

ALL MIGRAINES HAPPEN WHEN YOU ARE IN FIGHT-OR-FLIGHT MODE.

WHAT YOU NEED TO KNOW AS YOU HEAL FROM MIGRAINES

Hydrate, Hydrate, Hydrate

When you are getting a migraine or already have one, you cannot drink too much. What has likely happened is that your *fascia* (a web of connective tissue that interfaces with your muscles, organs, and cells throughout your body, storing water and fat tissue and providing a pathway for lymph, nerves, and blood vessels) has squeezed hydration out to help your brain. You need to replenish all that hydration, which can take a gallon or more. Drink as much as you can without making yourself ill. For most people, that means eight glasses of liquid, so drink up. The higher the quality of what you drink, such as coconut water, the less you will need to become hydrated. If you are urinating pale yellow and frequently, then you are likely hydrated.

Make hydration a priority to prevent migraines. Hydration is affected by what you eat, as well. Shift your diet away from dry foods and toward fresh vegetables and fruit. This will also help with your mineral balance.

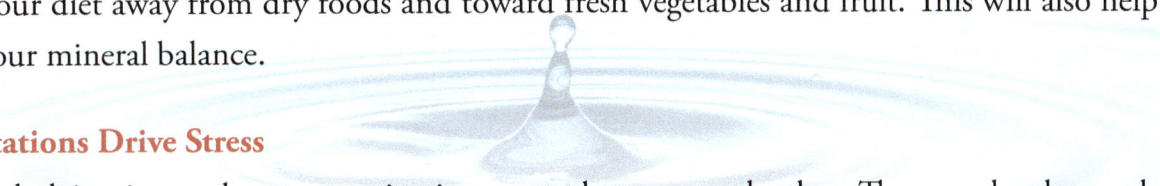

Expectations Drive Stress

The underlying issues that cause migraines can take years to develop. They can be the result of your habits and attitudes toward your life. Truly stopping migraines from developing may require time and a shift in your perspective.

Over the past two years, I have interviewed several women and a few men with migraines. I asked them to try the practice of *Stop, Drop, Roll, and Smile.* I told these headache sufferers to learn to recognize the early warning signs of a migraine coming on, and to stop for 20 minutes and give their brains and bodies the liquids, stretching, deep breathing, glucose, relaxation, and minerals that they need. I asked them to ground themselves (drop their awareness into their bodies), smile, enjoy a little satisfaction with life, and change their thoughts to positive ones.

I heard one message consistently, and I saw a very distinctive pattern among those who suffer from migraines.

Every person I spoke to said the same thing: "When I feel the early symptoms, I can't stop for 15 or 20 minutes. There is just no time." They also said their migraines came on at the worst times, when they had to meet a deadline or had another important meeting they could not miss.

Do you see the pattern? This pattern is often due to the body's addiction to hormones that are active when we are moving fast and working hard. Adrenaline is one of several hormone chemicals that we can become addicted to. If that happens, the body and brain don't want to stop activity because they want the constant flow of adrenaline, even when this is unhealthy. This is unconscious and difficult to override.

Consider a Perspective Shift

When the pressure is so great that you don't have 15 minutes for self-care, that is when the fight-or-flight response is the strongest. You have to perform (or you believe that you do), and that is like being chased by a lion. You can't stop and rest if a lion is chasing you.

This is a pattern consistent with those who suffer from migraines. The brain is locked into a thought process of *I can't stop or else something bad will happen* (i.e., get eaten by a lion, or their boss, or their spouse—or whatever their lion is).

You may think it is more important to finish the task at hand or finish a meeting rather than focus on your physical needs. To avoid the impending migraine, you must shift your mindset and tell yourself, "There is no lion. I am making up the lion." If your life consists of feeling as though lions are chasing you on a regular basis, consider making a change.

The irony is, if a migraine sufferer does not take a 20-minute break at the right moment, they will likely end up with a three-day migraine. Then, if they don't take harmful medications to cover up the pain, they will end up suffering in a dark room, getting nothing done.

HEALING TIP:
If you have any difficulty stopping immediately upon having early symptoms, be aware of this process and teach yourself that you perform at your best when you have what you need. Break the habit of prioritizing duty over taking care of your brain and body. You can make this shift with the thought that you are the person doing the work, so you are the priority since the job cannot be completed without you. This is a habit you can change.

MIGRAINE PRESCRIPTIONS CAN MAKE YOUR HEADACHES WORSE/ MORE FREQUENT

A 20-minute break or a few focused minutes of being present with your body could save you days of pain and a hangover from the pain. It could save your health from the harmful effects of the pharmaceutical drugs used to treat migraines. The truth is, long-term use of pharmaceutical drugs can become one of the causes of migraines as well as the cause of increased frequency of migraines.

LONG-TERM USE OF PHARMACEUTICAL DRUGS, INCLUDING MIGRAINE MEDICATIONS, CAN *CAUSE* MIGRAINES AND *INCREASE THE FREQUENCY* OF MIGRAINES.

When you are caught up in a lifestyle pattern that prevents you from keeping your body in balance, you are at risk for migraines or other health issues. If your body's ability to regulate blood flow is impaired by one or more causes, migraines can result.

ATTITUDES, HABITS, AND CONDITIONS THAT CAN CAUSE FIGHT-OR-FLIGHT MODE

Your thought patterns and expectations for yourself can throw your body out of balance. Emotional and physical stresses outside yourself can also throw you out of balance. In either case, the fix starts with you. You can reduce the current demands you place on yourself. You can work to recognize what situations are outside of your control, step back, and decide how to remove yourself from those stresses, rather than simply reacting to them.

As you review the list below, please remove *all* judgement about why you or anyone has these patterns. In the past, there has been too much judgement against those who suffer from migraines. There is no need or room for judgement—what you need is knowledge and healing. The fastest way to heal is to be gentle and kind to yourself and take the pressure and judgement away.

Do any of the following scenarios sound familiar to you? You may recognize more than one.

1. **Overachiever**: You push your body beyond its limits, draining the physical resources required for the brain to function. You may not be doing this intentionally or be aware of it when you do it. You may have a disconnect between your brain and your body and often ignore your body's needs. You are inside your head—not grounded (aware of your body) and not responding to your physical needs, such as food, water, rest, stretching, deep breathing, relaxation, etc. You may have less awareness of your body because of a head trauma, neck injury affecting the brain stem, or an emotional trauma. You may have self-imposed pressure to succeed at all costs, creating a feeling of heavy, demanding burdens. Perhaps you feel a need to please others or prove wor-

thiness. You are not taking time to smell the roses and be satisfied with life. You're in survival mode, pushing through, barely getting by, feeling that there is no time to rest and just do nothing. Many people live life in this mode. Not all of them get migraines.

2. **Anxiety:** You are in a pattern of going into fight or flight and getting stuck in a shallow breathing mode, directing resources to the muscles and away from the brain. Your body is releasing adrenaline and epinephrine hormones and you are low on serotonin. You don't relax and are always on guard, ready for whatever is coming next. You are prepared for the other shoe to drop, or an emergency to happen at any moment. You are productive and running from one task to the next. There is no time to slow down. Getting out of this repetition can prove to be challenging, because the pattern is very strong.

3. **Toxicity:** A common cause of recurring migraines is liver damage or neurotoxin exposure. These can be due to pharmaceutical drugs, alcohol, mold, or other toxins. Pain relievers and migraine medications add fuel to this fire and cause more migraines. In this situation, you may have had years of anti-inflammatory over-the-counter (OTC) or prescription drugs. These include Motrin or Advil. Perhaps you have taken codeine or other opiate pain relievers. You may be taking migraine medication, which causes further damage to the liver and blood vessels. Or, you have had a lot of alcohol or exposure to toxins and your liver is not working at its best. In the case of toxicity, your liver is not able to clean your blood of toxins and your blood vessels cannot deliver as much oxygen and nutrients to the brain as they should. If your liver damage is caused by ibuprofen, migraine meds, or other pain medication, chances are your blood vessels have some damage as well. Part of your healing will be to *stop* those medications.

4. **Head Injuries:** Head and neck injuries can underlie your migraine headaches. Impingements to vessels or nerves in your neck and head can cause your autonomic nerve system to react to this perceived threat by going into fight or flight. Part of your healing may be teaching your body that this is not a threat, if you can't resolve the impingement with the help of a specially trained physical therapist or other provider trained in soft tissue adjustments. If you have had one or more head or upper back injuries and/or whiplash, the stress-relieving activities listed in the bonus material will be especially important. This is also true if you have frequent neck pain and a tight jaw or pain at the base of your skull. Your long-term healing may require the assistance of a physical therapist, osteopath, or chiropractor. However, there is much you can do for yourself to promote proper alignment of the neck so that, over time, you won't need long-term care from a specialist to stay in alignment.

THE MIGRAINE LOOP

Any one of the behavioral patterns or conditions described above can keep what I call the *migraine loop* cycling, over and over. As the cycle fuels the growing fire of pain in your head, it gets worse and worse and spins out of control.

The migraine loop looks like this:

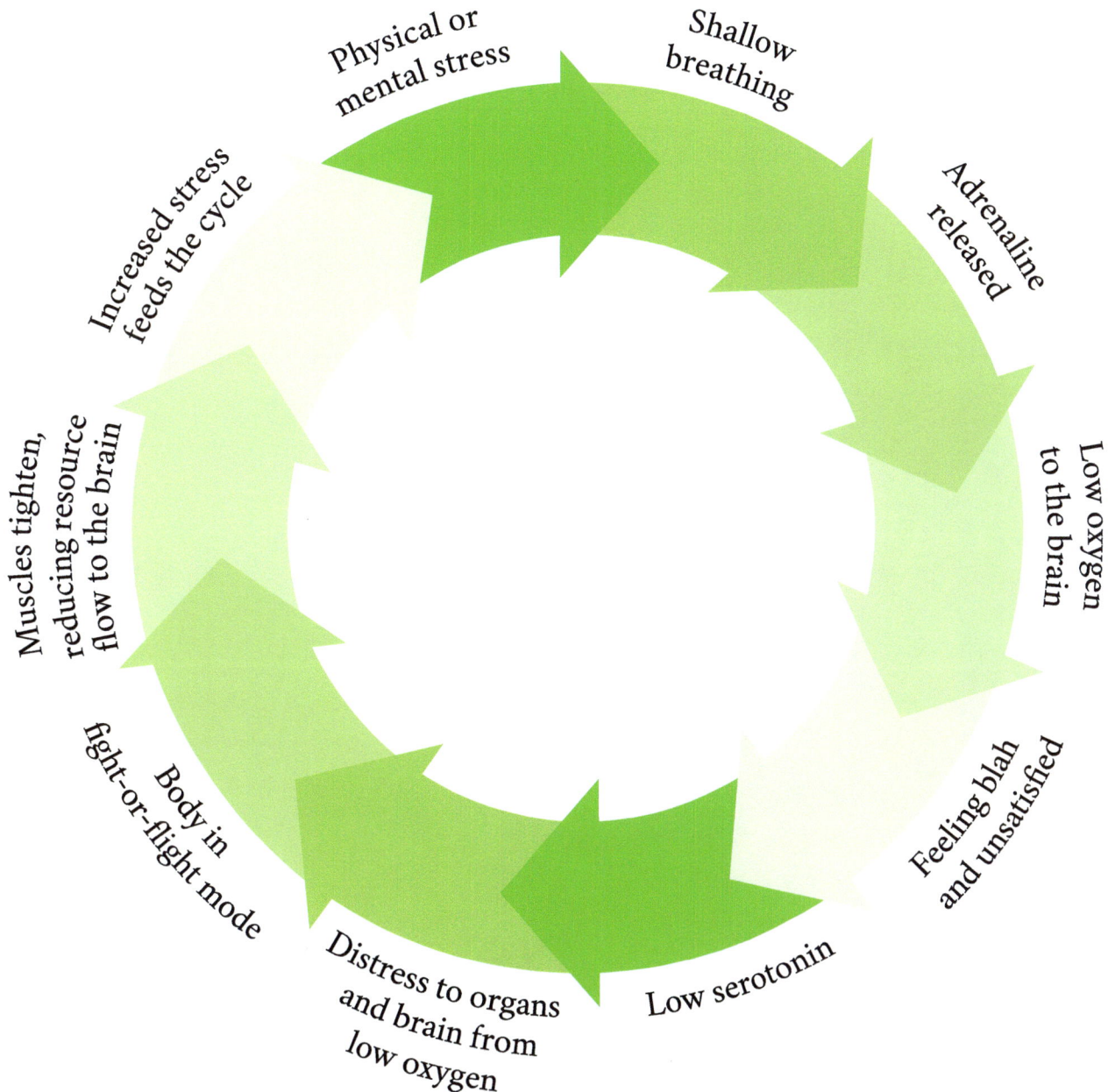

Physical or mental stress

Shallow breathing

Adrenaline released

Low oxygen to the brain

Feeling blah and unsatisfied

Low serotonin

Distress to organs and brain from low oxygen

Body in fight-or-flight mode

Muscles tighten, reducing resource flow to the brain

Increased stress feeds the cycle

Think of the stimulation to the nervous system as quantifiable, like a barometer that measures the number of neurons firing at any given moment. Since the neurons require resources, the number of neurons that can fire at any moment is dependent upon your current level of *homeostasis* (that is, the number of neurons supported by your current supply of resources—a sort of equilibrium).

If your body is unhealthy or dealing with a health condition affecting blood flow, or if you are low on hydration, glucose, and minerals, any of these conditions will limit your threshold for neurons that can fire. The stronger your body's ability to deliver resources to the nervous system, the more mental and emotional stimulation you can endure at any given time.

If your liver is toxic or your blood vessels are compromised, then your nervous system will have a lower threshold, triggering a migraine more easily than it would in a person with a better ability to deliver resources to the nervous system.

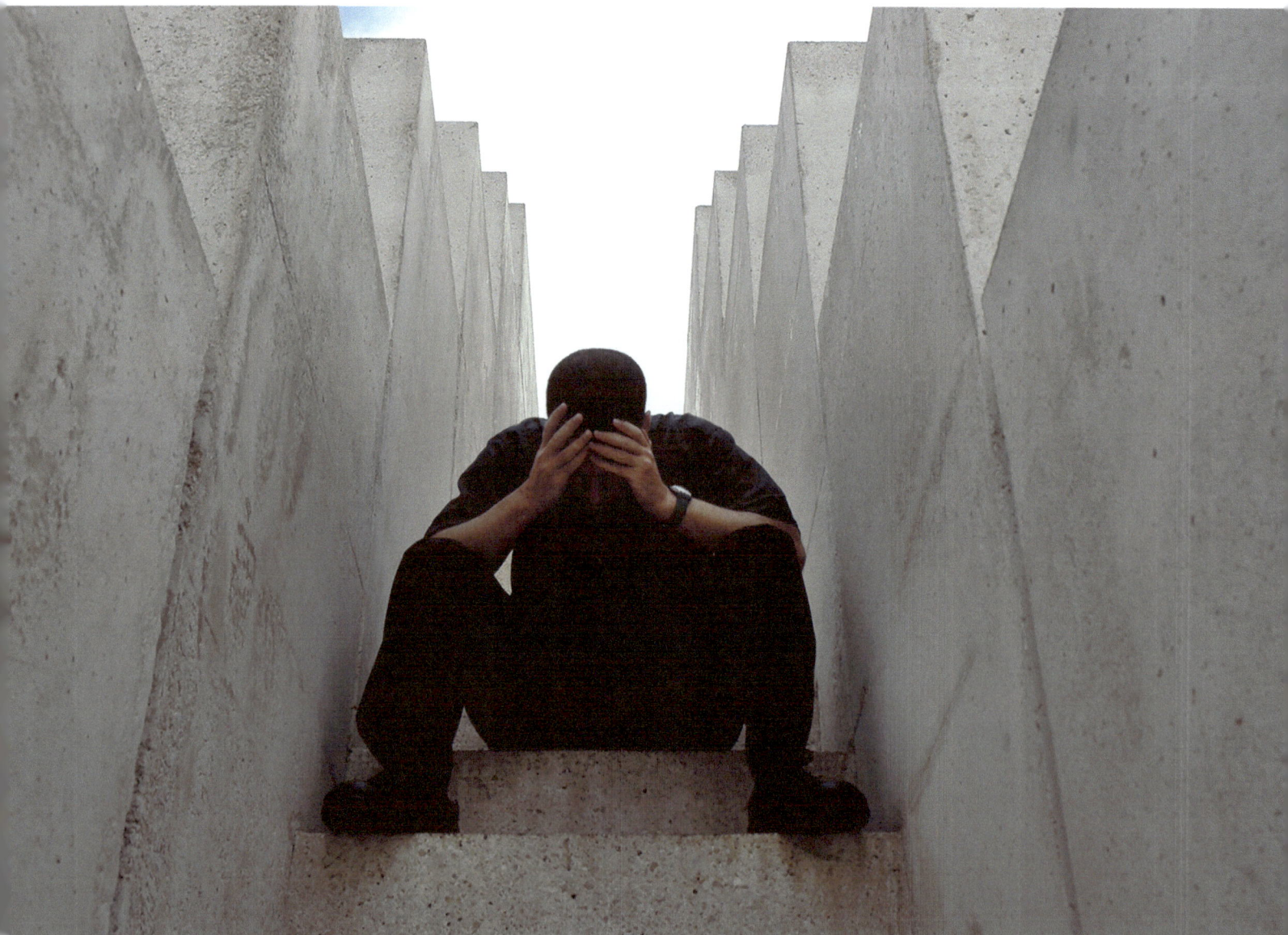

STEP 2:
DROP Your Breath and Your Awareness

WHAT TO DO RIGHT NOW

Once you have reduced nervous system stimulation, you need to drop your awareness into your belly and do a minimum of 10 minutes of *belly breathing*—expanding your diaphragm, relaxing your shoulders and jaw, pausing after a full inhale, and fully exhaling the breath to release all carbon dioxide from the lungs and blood. This will help you move to rest-and-digest mode.

DROP

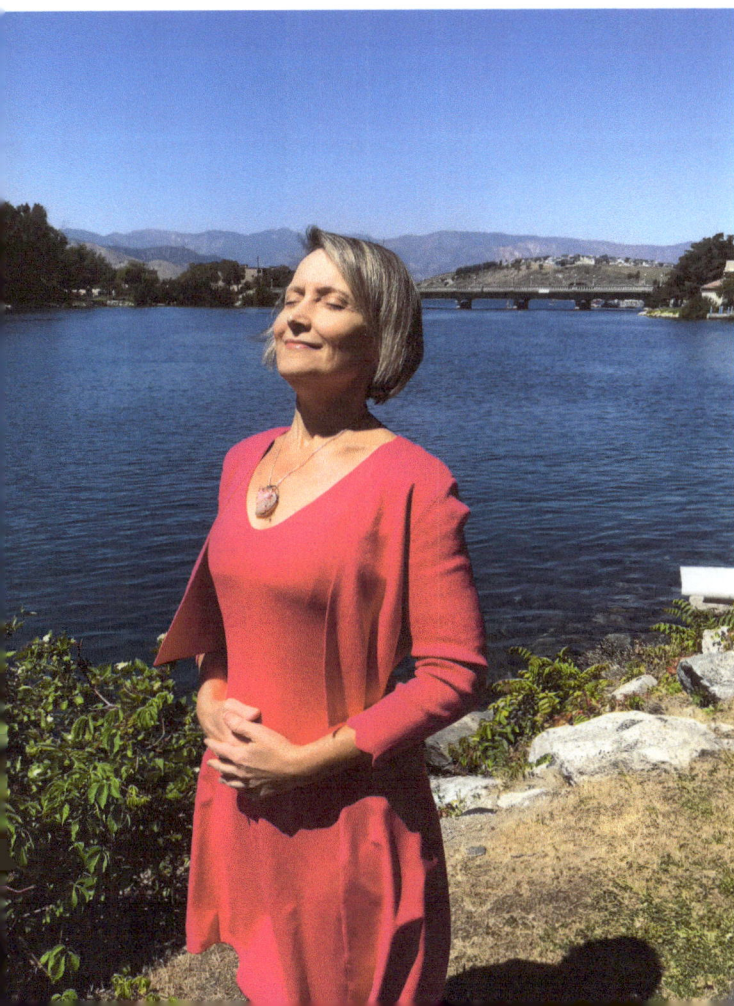

Try this right now: Notice your breath, very carefully. Take a few minutes. Notice how your chest or stomach moves when you breathe, and how long your inhale breaths are. Now pause after each inhale, and fully express all of the air in your lungs. Keep exhaling until you can't exhale any more. Repeat this for several breaths.

When you are in a state of rest and digest, your breathing is relaxed and you feel calm, at ease. There is a feeling of satisfaction and content.

After five minutes, notice your breath again. Every time your breath deepens and begins from expanding the diaphragm, more oxygen is delivered to the body and it calms the nervous system. Try adding a big sigh on the exhale with a sound. AAhhhhh!

WHAT YOU NEED TO KNOW AS YOU HEAL FROM MIGRAINES

Unfortunately, people can literally get stuck in fight or flight and try as they might, they can't seem to change their state. One way that can work efficiently and effectively to make this transition is to focus on your breathing and control it, so that you take deep breaths and fully exhale them. If focused breathing does not help you to transition into rest and digest, then you may have a strong, well-established pattern of stress that your body is accustomed to, or even addicted to. In this case, you may need more time and possibly a nap, deep stretching or massage, or other forms of deep relaxation to calm down and sooth the nervous system.

YOUR EXHALES SHOULD TAKE LONGER THAN YOUR INHALES FOR EFFECTIVE, DEEP BELLY BREATHING TO CALM YOUR SYSTEM.

Dropping your breath means expanding your diaphragm to draw air deep into your lower lungs. Stress causes you to breathe shallowly. When you are relaxed, you breathe into the lower chambers of your lungs. This is part of resting and healing. Anytime you need to heal your body, breathe into the lower chambers of the lungs with the help of your diaphragm.

If a migraine is coming on, you are not properly using your diaphragm to breathe deeply, slowly, and calmly.

IT TAKES EFFORT TO MAKE NEW HABITS

Learning to breathe deeply as your "normal" is not as easy as it sounds. When I began to get well, I knew what I had to do was stop, drop, roll, and smile at the very first signs of a migraine. I would stop what I was doing at work and get present with my body.

I would lie down to breathe slowly, and I often found I couldn't breathe in a relaxed way. Even with conscious effort and no other activity, I couldn't slow down my breath and release the tension to expand my diaphragm consistently. I was in a pattern of resistance and tension.

I could not figure out how to shift this pattern. I applied effort and focus, with poor results. I had allowed circumstances in my life to cause me to hold my body tightly. When I learned to exhale consistently longer than I inhaled, to fully express the carbon dioxide, I finally could relax my muscles enough to breathe easy. This usually worked.

Breathing shallowly causes a buildup of carbon dioxide in the lungs and blood stream. This buildup can lock you into a stressed state. To move out of the stressed state, you need to fully exhale to push out the carbon dioxide.

When you exhale longer breaths than you inhale, you stimulate the rest and digest state of the nervous system. Until you are breathing in a calm, relaxed state, you will remain locked in stress and distress, even when there is no threat.

The HeartMath Institute (www.HeartMath.org) discovered through years of research that the inhalation breath stimulated the fight-or-flight mode and the exhalation stimulated rest and digest.

Shallow breathing is enough of a threat to limit resources to the nervous system in a person who already has an out-of-balance system. Calm, slow breathing is critical to a pain-free head. Belly breathing communicates to the *vagus nerve* that all is well.

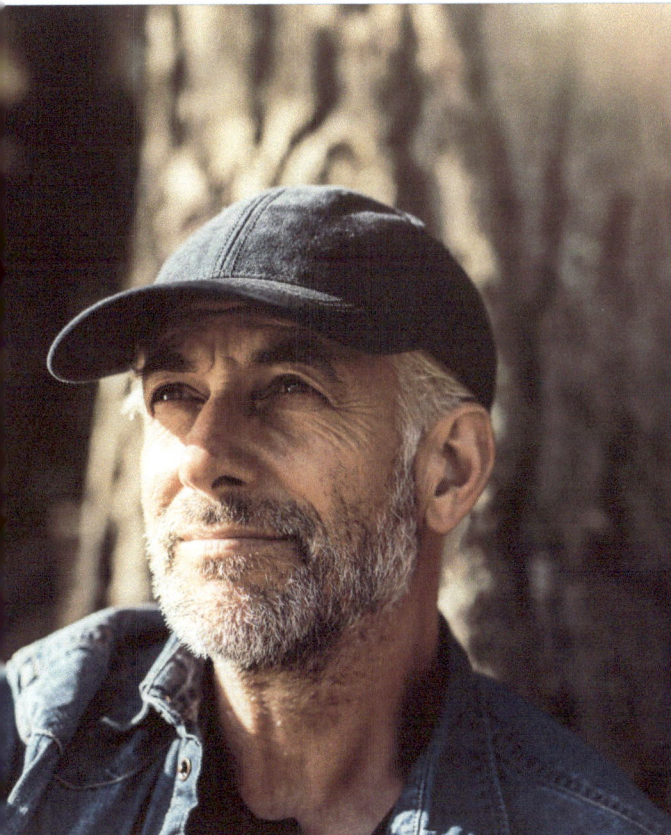

EXHALING FULLY ALSO HELPS THE BODY INHALE MORE AIR BY EXPANDING THE DIAPHRAGM. SIMPLY TAKING FIVE MINUTES FOR LONG, SLOW EXHALES CAN SHIFT THE NERVOUS SYSTEM.

The vagus nerve is the longest of the 12 cranial nerve pairs, connecting the neck, heart, lungs, and abdomen to the brain. It communicates that all is well to the autonomic nervous system—and it also communicates when all is *not* well.

Healing Tip: Get into a habit of becoming aware of your breath several times throughout the day. Check to see if your chest moves with each breath or if you are using your diaphragm correctly. Your chest should not move significantly. Relax your breath as needed. Practice correct breathing while sitting and walking. Make a habit of being aware of your body and how you are breathing. Over time, you will become more conscious and this will help you find your balance before a problem can begin. It will also promote body healing.

LEARNING TO CONNECT BODY AND MIND

Drop also means being present with your body and responding to the signals it gives you. The awareness between mind and body is an ever-growing union, a dance for two. If you have migraines, the dance is not in sync. You are missing your steps and your communication is breaking down—the mind/body relationship is off balance, and the result is disease. You can repair this relationship with baby steps and awareness. The HeartMath Institute has created a device that helps you monitor your mind/body connection with immediate biofeedback to stay in balance. Visit RealMigraineSolutions.com for more about the HeartMath Institute's feedback device.

Healing Tip: Develop a habit of checking in with your body throughout the day. Notice which areas of your body tend to get tight when you have any stress. Start with your feet. Think about relaxing your feet. Take a few breaths with your awareness on your feet. Wiggle them and breathe. Once your feet are relaxed, move your awareness to your ankles and calves and relax them. Most people will notice that tension begins in their feet and moves up the body, culminating at the neck and head. If you keep your feet relaxed, the rest of your body will follow.

Over time, the mind/body connection becomes effortless and whole—one energy—one smooth, flowing circuit. The nervous system knows when you need to rest and digest, when you need fight or flight, and how to tune everything else out for a little one-on-one dance of pure bliss, love, and appreciation for each other. It's the perfect marriage, but it takes practice.

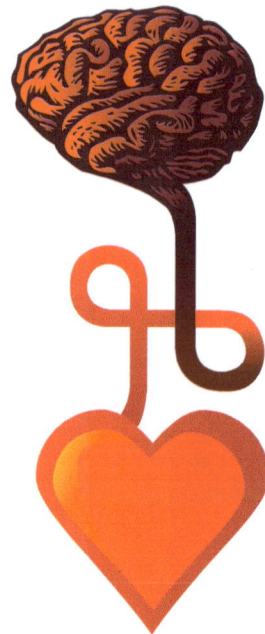

Computers have made it easy to break the bond of mind and body. We spend our days using an instrument that requires holding our bodies in an unnatural position. Some jobs don't use a computer but require repetitive motion, causing the same kind of tension. Many of us must retrain the communication and presence between mind and body.

The people you know who work all day at a computer and don't get migraines have trained their mind and body to communicate, or breathe properly and don't get into fight or flight, or suffer from a different ailment due to that stress. If the communication is lacking, their bodies will develop health issues, depending on their weaknesses. They might develop lethargy, sleep issues, chronic back pain, or depression—and the list goes on. If their feedback loop is broken, a disease will develop.

For those with migraines, there is a propensity for head pain due to many factors. I have identified five underlying causes for migraine headaches, through my own experiences and research. I have described and addressed them in my book *The Migraine Protocol,* for long-term healing and freedom from migraine pain. You cannot achieve this by simply taking prescription medications. I had all five of the causes of migraines—and my joy in finding healing is what I truly want to share with you.

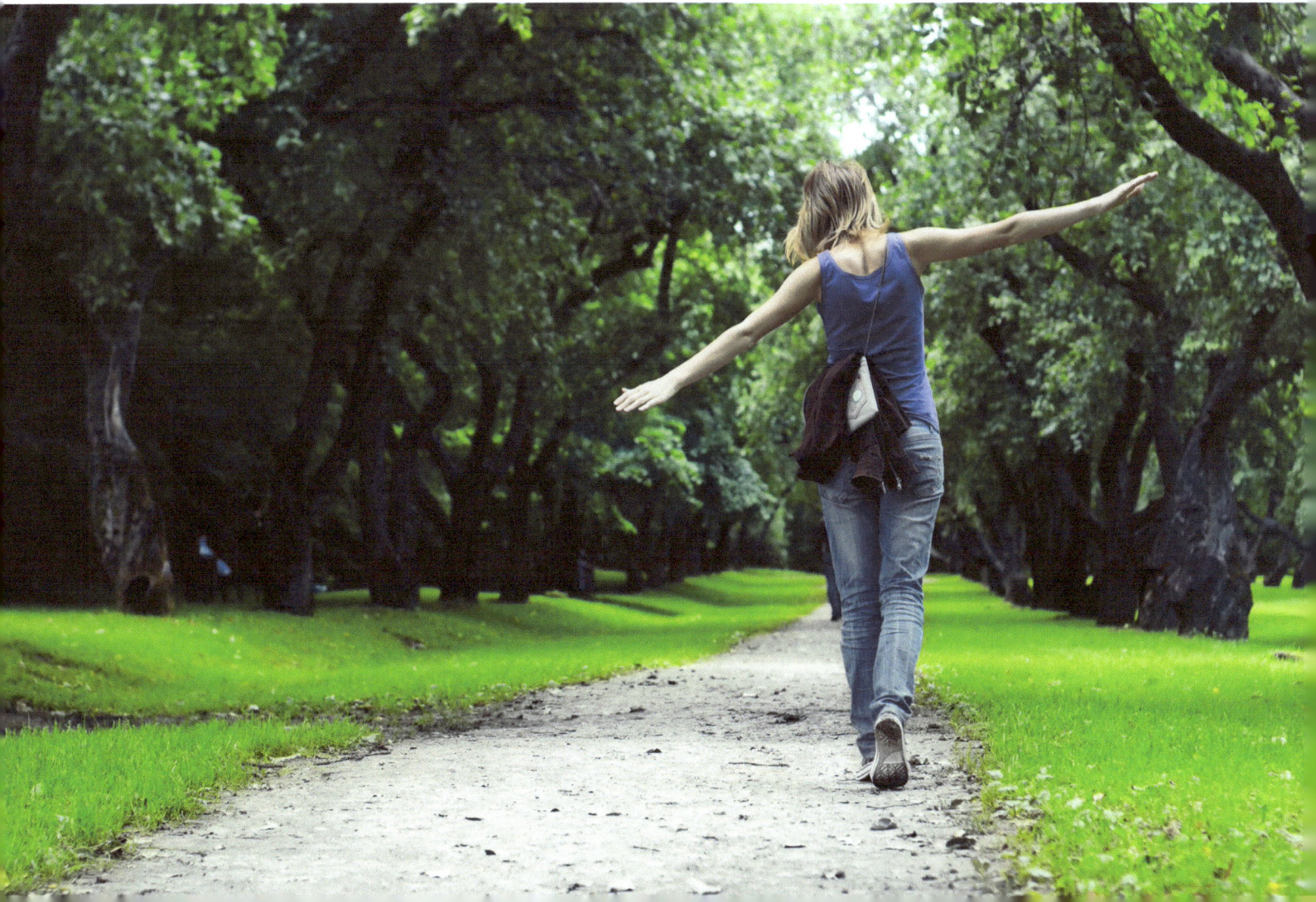

RELAXING AND GROUNDING YOURSELF SLOWS DOWN THE CONSUMPTION OF RESOURCES AND DIRECTS THEM TO THE NERVOUS SYSTEM.

STEP 3:
ROLL Out the Fascia

In the earliest stages of a migraine, you can quickly ward it off by *grounding* yourself and being present with your body. This act slows down the consumption of resources and directs them to the nervous system. Additionally, you can replenish the required resources to help calm the nervous system. Grounding your energy will release good hormones and can shift your body from fight or flight into rest and digest.

ROLL

WHAT TO DO RIGHT NOW

1. Relax your fascia and muscles: The following have worked for me and others. Find the method that works best for you.

- Relax your jaw, shoulders, and neck. Practice good posture and feel the muscles relax in your back and shoulders.

- Undulate your spine so that the spinal fluid can reach your brain and spinal nerves as it should.

- Release the tension in your muscles.

- Use a foam roller.

- Get a back and/or neck massage.

- Lie down and rest your neck and jaw.

- Use all-natural muscle relaxing creams and oils (see the list in the Resources section and at RealMigraineSolutions.com)

- Do long, slow, gentle stretches to allow time for the fascia to relax and release tension.

The fascia, muscles, and many systems in your body are connected.[4] The fascia can account for up to 20 percent of your body's mass.[5] Relaxing your muscles and fascia helps to put your body into rest-and-digest mode.

For effective relaxation, hydration and minerals are also required, which were covered in the first step, Stop. Find what works best for you and adopt that as your method for the Roll part of this process. We are all unique and you need to find the way to relax your muscles that works best for you.

2. Ground yourself: Grounding is one more way to shift your body out of fight-or-flight mode. You can ground yourself relatively easily with a few simple steps.

Nature gave us simple ways to heal and balance the body. These steps are so valuable that their simple nature should not be overlooked.

- Become *present* in the moment—what is happening with your body and surroundings. Do this in a nonjudgmental way, with a focus on the positive.
- Walk barefoot on the earth. This immediately releases electrical energy from your body and balances the electrical impulses. This is one reason why a walk on the beach feels so good. If it is cold outside, this is difficult to do, but a walk in nature will help, or touching a plant, rock, or animal helps to release this overcharge.
- Have another person who is grounded touch you or be present with you. They are assisting you because their circuits are already grounded and they are now focusing on you.
- Essential oils, flowers, and natural fragrances such as herbs and spices are all very grounding.

Try any of the above techniques and then release a big sigh to expel carbon dioxide and feel a sense of peace and calm.

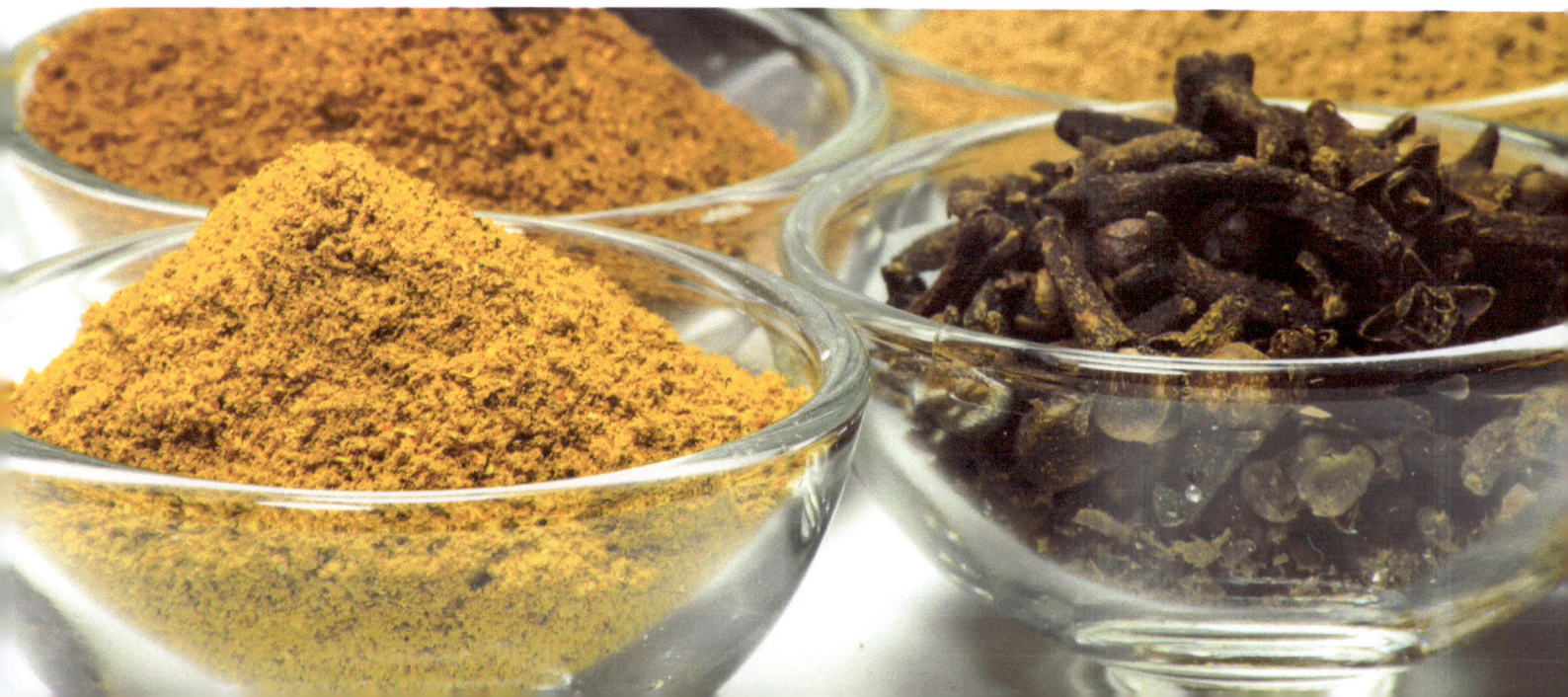

WHAT YOU NEED TO KNOW AS YOU HEAL FROM MIGRAINES

Fascia, Muscles, and Hydration

Once you are in the early stages of a migraine, you are likely experiencing tension, which may not be noticeable. Tension can be found and felt anywhere in the body because the *fascia* surrounds and connects every cell.

Your muscles cannot relax without relaxing the fascia. The fascia must relax first. It takes time, and long, slow, gentle stretches work best with deep, slow breathing. Undulating the spine helps increase circulation of blood, nerve signals, and the lymph and spinal fluids to help with full-body communication.

Also, the fascia requires proper hydration to function optimally. Dehydration affects every cell in the body in more ways than one, but certainly by affecting the fascia and nervous system. Medical scientists believe the fascia can hold up to four gallons of water. When you are sufficiently hydrated and have the right balance of minerals, the fascia can soak up or release hydration as needed.

A TIGHT FASCIA GREATLY AFFECTS A MIGRAINE. IT REDUCES THE FLOW OF *ALL* RESOURCES.

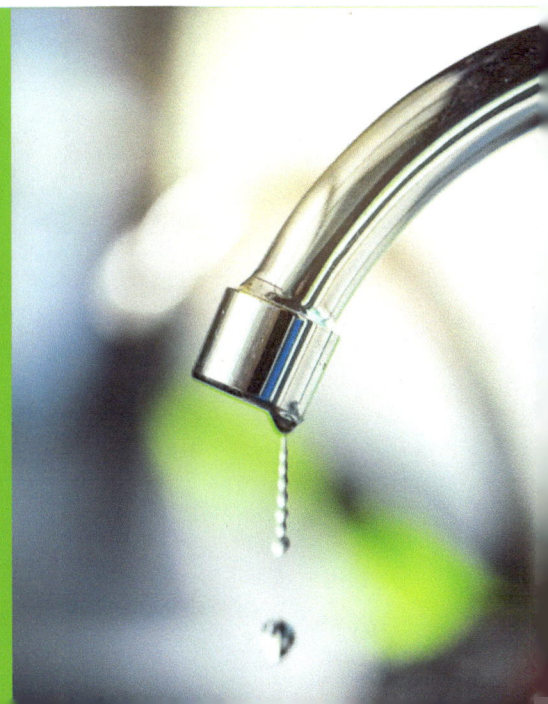

The fascia acts like a sponge, holding water. If the brain needs more hydration, the fascia can "squeeze" hydration out of its spongy fibers to send to the brain. This action helps the brain for short-term relief. However, this moisture must also be replenished. Squeezing moisture out of the fascia can cause the fascia to become tight from lack of fluids, and then muscle fibers also become tight.

Stretching, massage, hydration, movement, deep breathing, and relaxation all help a tight fascia to release its grip. Fascia does not release quickly. It is a highly complex fabric designed to protect the body and hold it together. Without the fascia, you would be a glob of bones and tissue, unable to move. The fascia gives your body its shape and enables the muscles, tendons, and bones to work together.

Healing Tip:
Your brain functions on electrical charges, similar to electricity. When the brain is firing a lot, it gets hot. Spinal fluid and oxygen cool off the brain and keep the electrical charges from overheating. Sitting at a computer and breathing shallow can cause the brain to get too hot, causing pain or the feeling of a hot head. Moving the spinal fluid is one way to cool off your brain during high intellectual activity.

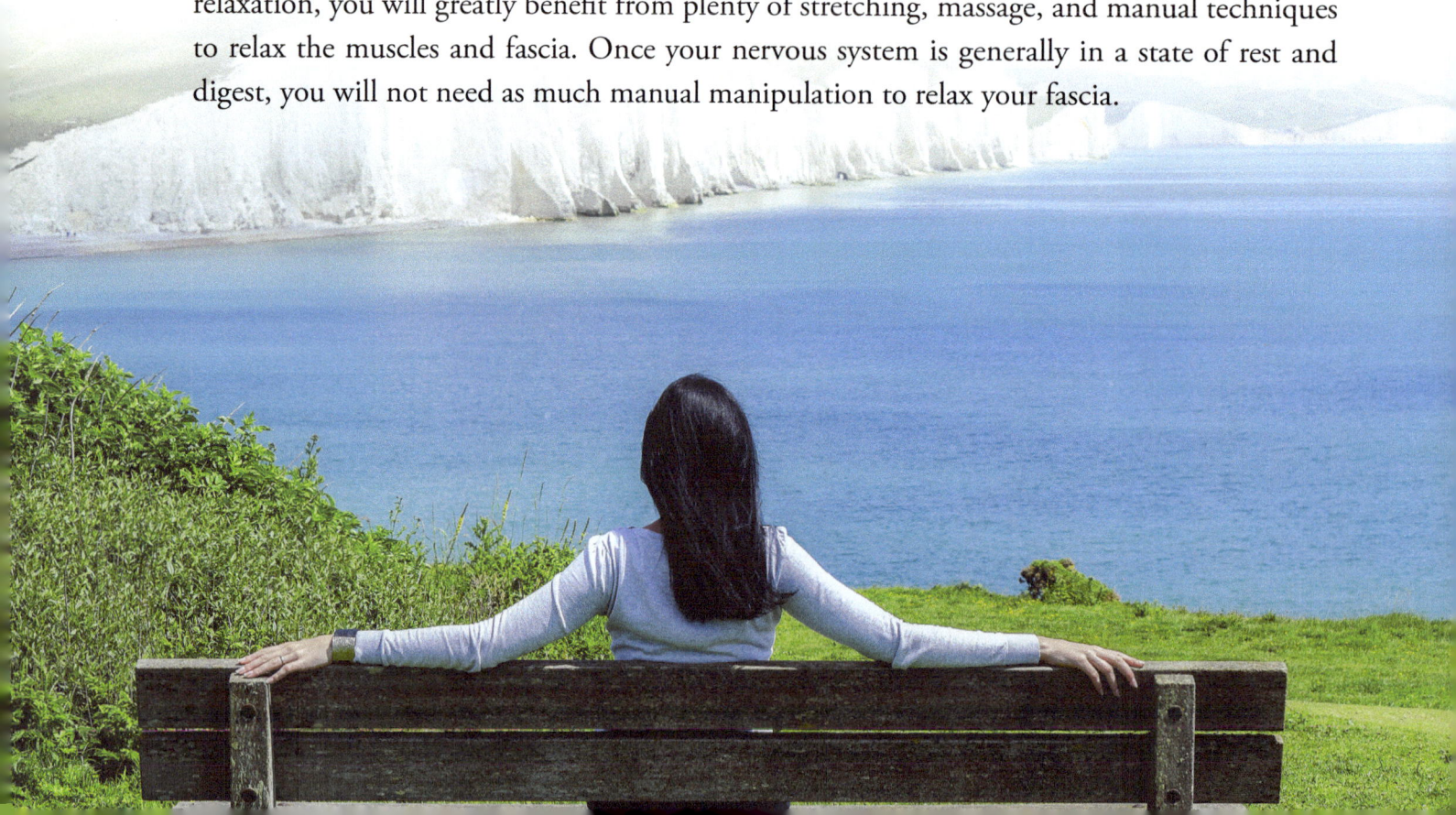

When you are relaxed, your fascia is functioning optimally, as are all your body systems. Relaxation accompanies certain emotions and chemicals. Until you enjoy a lifestyle of frequent relaxation, you will greatly benefit from plenty of stretching, massage, and manual techniques to relax the muscles and fascia. Once your nervous system is generally in a state of rest and digest, you will not need as much manual manipulation to relax your fascia.

GROUNDING

To relax more quickly, you must *ground* the nervous system. The fastest way to ground is to become fully present with your body and feel a sense of satisfaction with life. When you ground the electrical system of your body, the nervous system works optimally and it goes into rest and digest. It no longer feels a threat and stops depleting the resources required by the brain and central nervous system.

What Is Grounding?

You may have heard the term "to be grounded," but what does that mean? Grounding, also called *earthing,* is a term related to the electricity vernacular. In effect, it means to keep the electrical impulses of the nervous system in balance. When you experience stress, or overthinking and overworking, your central nervous system fires a lot of signals. Those signals are electricity. Left unchecked, that electrical energy shoots through the body and brain and can increase in amperage (current). Grounding gives that electricity a way to release the buildup and bring the electrical system of the nervous system back into balance.

Physical stress can create a similar increase in current from the overfiring of nerves during body trauma. Grounding is valuable in calming the electrical impulses to avoid or stop the overfiring.

SIMPLE GROUNDING EXERCISE

Imagine you have time to lie in the cool grass, on a comfortable blanket under a big elm tree on a warm summer day. You close your eyes and ***drop*** your breath and awareness into the moment and the world around you. You feel the ground beneath you. The birds are singing and you hear the leaves rustle in the soft breeze.

You are breathing slowly, relaxed and calm, with no place to go. You don't have a thought in your head about how much time you have to lie there. You completely enjoy each moment as it comes. The temperature is so perfect you could fall asleep in the welcoming, fresh air. You inhale the fragrance from lilacs nearby. The breeze caresses your skin ever so gently.

As you notice all of this, you are fully present and you are not judging it. You are not thinking the lilacs should smell more like roses or the birds could sing more in harmony. You are taking it in, grateful for what exists around you. You are noticing, and the world is delivering sensations to you.

This is a feedback loop, with your consciousness noticing the physical world. It is the perfect balance of two polar energies, physical and consciousness. It's a beautiful exchange. The earth is feeding your energy and you appreciate how wonderful it all feels.

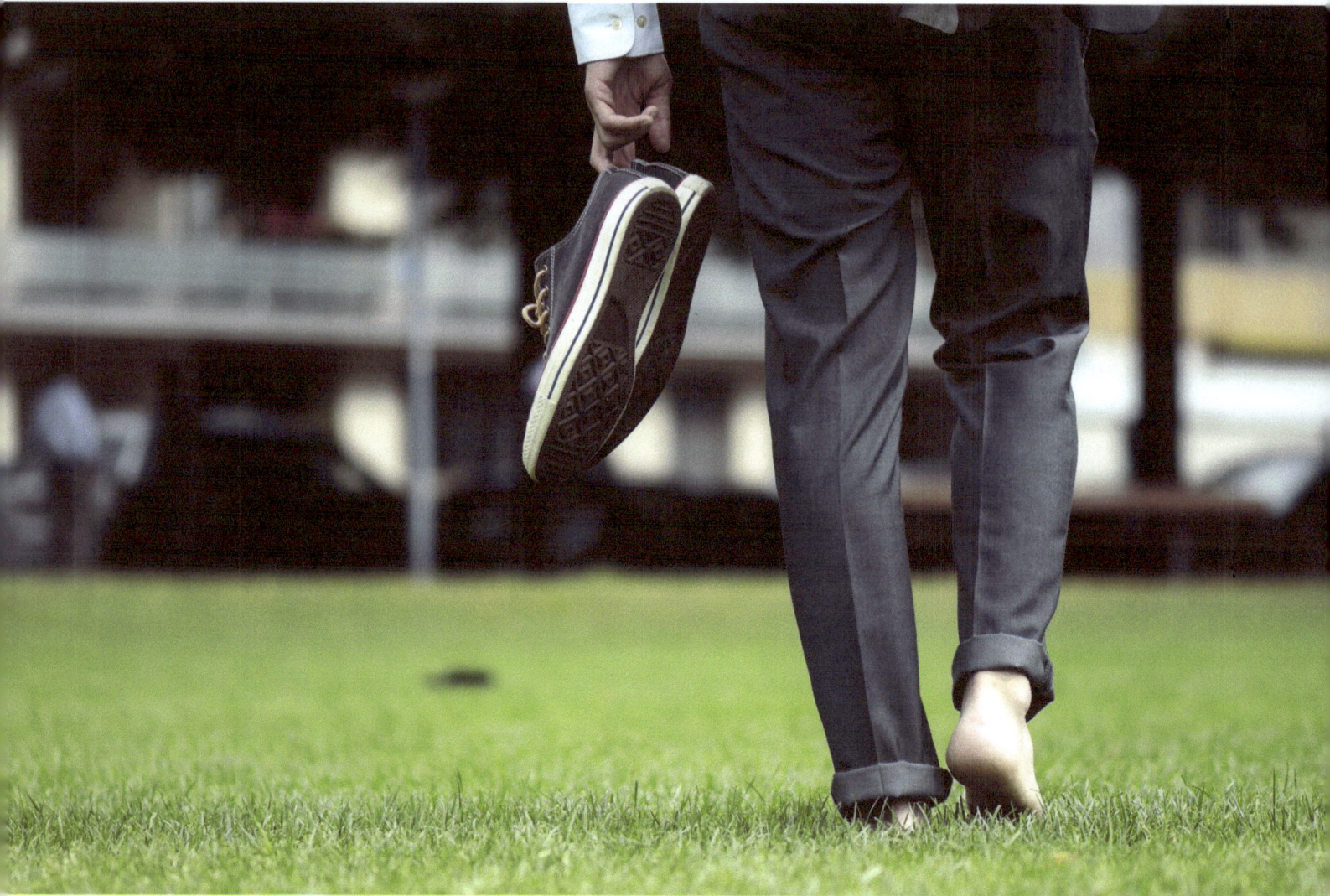

As you become more grounded, the nervous system knows things are getting better. When you accept the moment without resistance, healthy chemical signals such as the hormone serotonin are released, which relax the nervous system. Your breathing relaxes without your even being aware of it. More oxygen is directed to the brain, glucose and hydration are no longer directed to the muscles, and the nervous system can get more of what it needs.

You can create healthy habits that keep you grounded every day, by taking time to be present and not judge what is happening. Just notice, observe. Be with the moment as it occurs instead of being stuck in a thought pattern or cycle you can't release. When the peripheral nervous system is relaxed, pain signals subside.

In summary, *Roll*, stretch, hydrate, become present with the body, and relax the fascia and therefore muscles. Undulate the spine to roll the spinal fluid up to the brain. Roll the body to relax it.

STEP 4:
SMILE

When a migraine is beginning, many things happen with the brain and body. During this stressed state, cortisol and adrenaline are present in abundance, which signals to the brain and body, "All hands on deck! We have a problem."

This warning system works great for temporary issues. Long term, it wreaks havoc. One of those long-term effects can be migraine pain. To stop a migraine, you must direct more resources to your brain and calm the nervous system. If this sounds similar to Step 2, Drop, and 3, Roll, you are correct. Each of the four steps in this program is designed to achieve the same result—to move your body into a relaxed, rest-and-digest state. Migraines don't happen when you are in rest and digest.

SMILE

Our bodies have many layers of systems and feedback mechanisms related to relaxation and the fight-or-flight mode. To make the transition from fight or flight to rest and digest, you will shift (change) the chemicals that are pumping throughout your body.

WHAT TO DO RIGHT NOW

Smile: Smiling is one of the fastest ways to shift the chemicals in your body, but it needs to be genuine. To generate an authentic smile, think of something you are sincerely grateful for in your life. This could be as simple as having hands and feet that work, eyes that see, a family, or a pet. No matter what your life is like, you have something or someone you can appreciate. Appreciation is the secret sauce to happy hormones and therefore a good flow of energy, blood, and oxygen in your body.

Have you seen someone smile who is not happy? You know instantly that it's not authentic. Picture a fake smile or try to make one yourself. Fake smiles do not release happy hormones. In fact, they do the opposite. So the real trick is thinking of things that make you feel like smiling a true, authentic smile.

Appreciation in the present moment creates a feeling of love—for many people, this is the most powerful positive emotion. Being in love with life is appreciating your life right now, the way it is, and being grateful for it. Nothing tells the nervous system all is well like an appreciation for being alive.

WHAT YOU NEED TO KNOW AS YOU HEAL FROM MIGRAINES

Find Simple Joy in Your Life

Stress comes in the form of worry (mental), fear (emotional), and pinched nerves (physical). Many things can cause duress, but did you know that a lack of pleasure and joy can also? Lack of joy or satisfaction causes stress chemicals to be released. Shallow breathing follows, then the fascia tightens, slowing circulation throughout the body, and then you go into flight-or-flight mode. This redirects blood away from the brain. It also causes your muscles to become even tighter, squeezing hydration out of cells to help blood and oxygen flow, causing the fascia to tighten more, and this cycle repeats until it eventually shuts down the system. I described this earlier as a *migraine loop*.

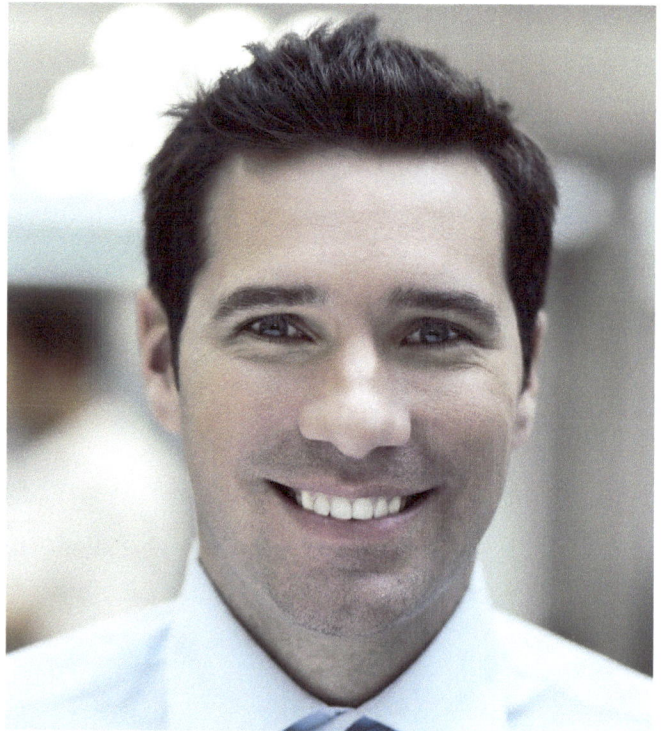

Good Thoughts = Good Health

Your thoughts and emotions about your life affect which chemicals are flowing in your body. Thought patterns determine where the body will become diseased and which area of the fascia will tighten up and where the body will suffer. For people who suffer from migraines, the jaw, upper neck, and upper back get the tightest. For people with a lot of stress but no migraines, perhaps the fascia of the stomach area gets tight, which doesn't cause them to get migraines.

Instead, it causes stomach and digestive issues. For others, it is the low back. It could be the feet, knees, or heart. It varies for each person. Learning the art of relaxing the fascia will stave off all kinds of health issues, not just migraines.

You can control the chemicals released in your body in order to feel a sense of relaxation, satisfaction, ease, peace, or joy. You can choose emotions that trigger chemical releases to relax the body, release serotonin, and allow the blood to flow to your head. When the happy hormones release, they chase away the stress hormones. It is as simple as *Stopping* what you are doing to feel joy and satisfaction. Life is meant to be joyful.

When you work all day without stopping to enjoy life, you will create body tension. Once you notice you are tight, you need to stop immediately, become *present,* and pay attention to the physical world, including your body.

Choose a Life You Enjoy

Sometimes people unknowingly resist life by being unhappy with what is happening. This stops love and well-being from flowing through you. When you don't want to do something, but you do it to please someone, to look good, or because you lack confidence to say no, you create resistance. An example is if your spouse wants to watch TV every night and you don't; you want to take night classes, but instead you sit and watch TV, hating it the whole time. Or you stay in a relationship despite abuse and decide that you don't have a choice. Migraines can be a sign that you have given up on your hopes and dreams and resigned yourself to put up with life instead of enjoying it.

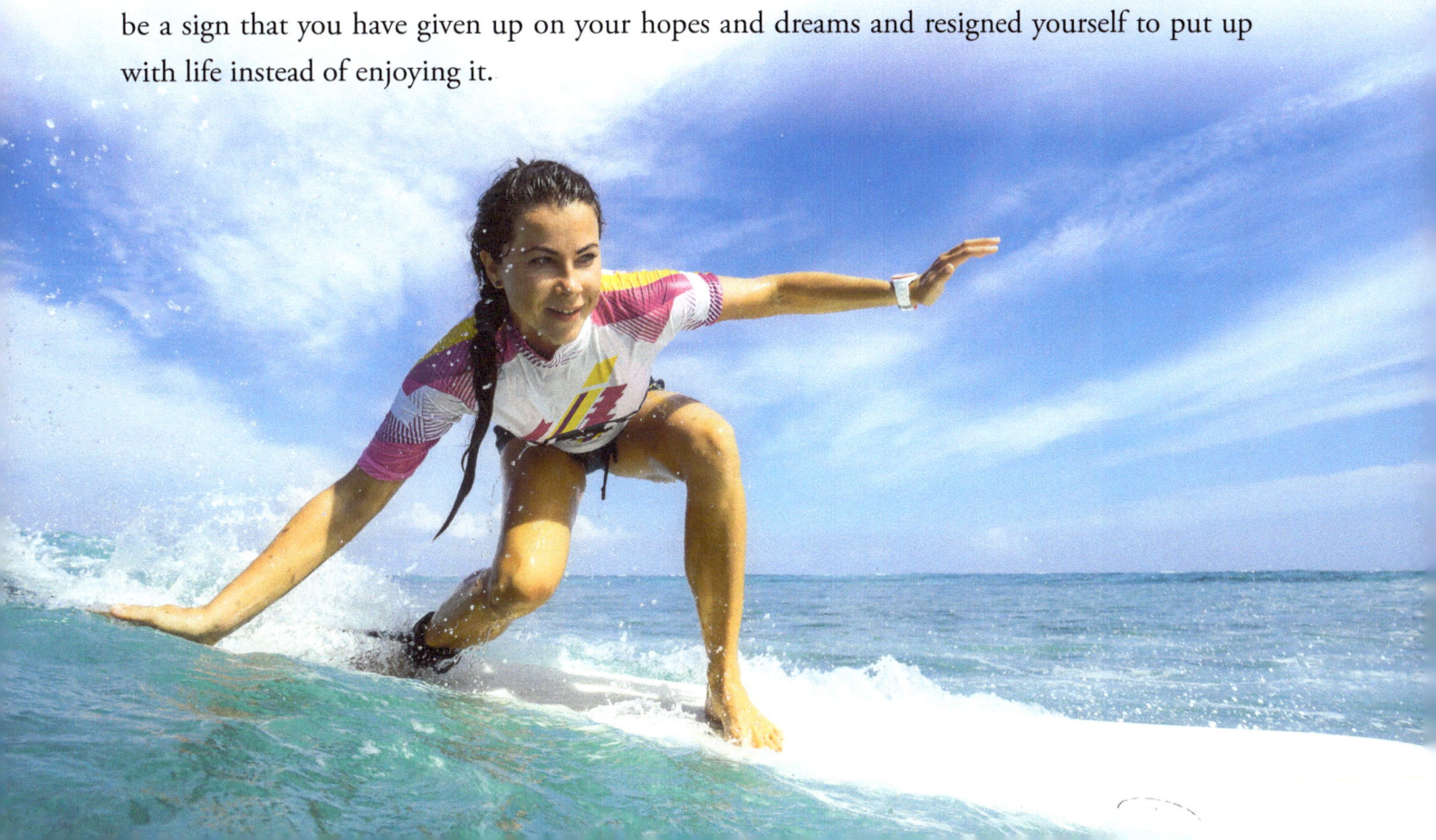

Find a Way to Deal With Grief and Loss

Sometimes resistance can be caused through trauma or grief; something terrible happened. If your migraines started following such an event, you may need help to come to terms with what has happened and learn to move forward in peace.

When you let love for life flow, free of all resistance, things work out. When you "feel the love" present in every creation, every creature, and every breath of air, even though this world can be chaotic and violent, you can see love is ever-present.

Remove Feelings of Resistance

When you tune in and "feel the love," you allow the fullness of who you are flow through you. Resistance does not allow this flow. Resistance feels like anger, frustration, dissatisfaction, depression, or guilt. It is being overwhelmed, lacking confidence, trying to meet others' expectations, or being a victim. Any of these situations and emotions can cause you pain.

Living a life to please others does not allow you to be who you are, nor does it allow your energy to flow naturally. This creates resistance, much like a resistor lowers the amperage in a circuit board. Too much resistance to the life you are living is like many resistors in one circuit board; eventually the amperage is too low to run the operations. The way to make the circuit energy flow is to feel love, joy, satisfaction, and positive emotions, which remove the resistance.

Find Your "Zone": The Mind-Body Dance

When you are satisfied and experiencing pleasure, you are aligned with the greater purpose of your life—you are happy. It is the opposite of resistance and the opposite of migraines. This is love flowing to and through you, and miracles can happen. It feels amazing to tune into this love or joy.

What causes you to feel complete joy? Some people think of it as getting in the "zone."

Basketball players, surfers, ballet dancers, actors, skateboarders, skiers, and painters all get this kind of elation from being fully present with their task at hand. They get into the "zone" and feel joy in the present moment— the world goes away. This creates a

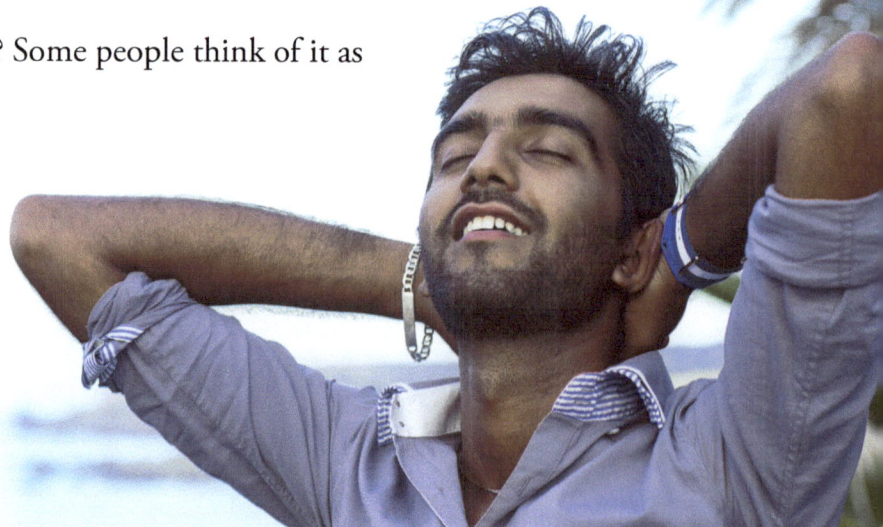

delicious feedback loop with a synergistic field of consciousness and the physical; your mind and body are working in one smooth, sensual dance. Nothing else matters in that moment.

What does the mind-body dance do for you?

1.   **Creates an open heart—turns your heart on**

2.   **Brings you into the moment**

3.   **Allows you to dance smoothly with the world around you**

4.   **Helps blood and electrical circulation flow freely**

If the mind-body dance you create involves joy, pleasure, or human touch, or you are touching the earth's surface with your feet or body, then you are becoming more grounded.

There are many ways to increase joy and satisfaction. What works for you may be different from anyone else. Here are some ideas to consider for increasing your enjoyment of your life:

1.   Accept or allow what is happening and smile with genuine appreciation for being alive. (In this case, it's good to fake it until you make it. If you are in pain, feel gratitude for the life you live when you don't have pain.)

2.   Recognize you do have control over how you feel, who you live with, where you work, how you spend your resources, and what you do in your free time. Victimhood steals away your life.

3.   Appreciate everything the way it is, free of any judgement about it or expectations from it, and take responsibility for your actions, feelings, and choices.

4.   Embrace life and feel a sense of satisfaction or love. This causes serotonin to release and the nerves to rest.

5.   Notice what is good about something and feel grateful, for that is a form of love.

6.   Let go of resistance to the world around you.

Healing Tip: If you can smile and pretend for a short length of time that all is well, perfect, and smooth in your world—if you can convince the brain there is nothing to worry about and everything is as it should be—the body and brain get a break from stress. Even if you don't believe it right now, fake it. Pretend all is well so you can experience that feeling. Over time you can find more and more moments of calm and bliss to enjoy and give the mind a break. The mind needs breaks from stress and worry. Take that break, even if it doesn't feel possible.

7. Stay present with your body and environment.

8. Breathe. Breath is your energy and life force. Feeling love requires joy, which begets breath and more life force.

Keep serotonin in flow by living a satisfied life with gratitude and by being fully present. This keeps your nervous system out of fight-or-flight mode.

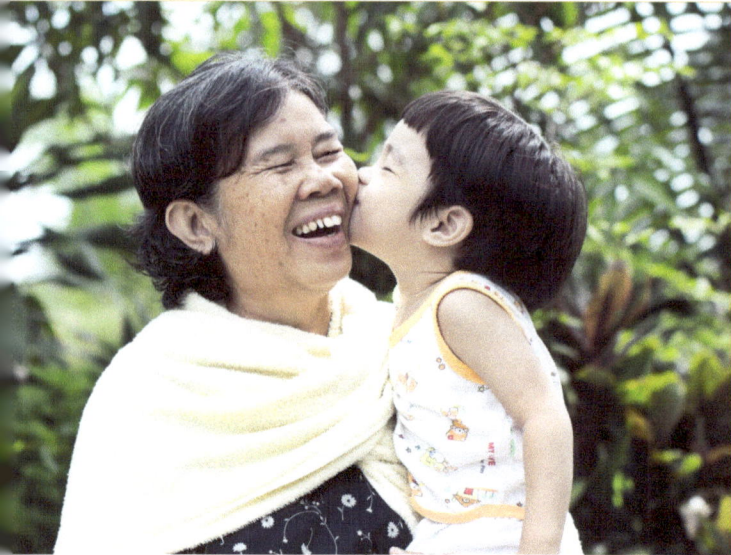

PREVENTING MIGRAINES IS PREVENTING THE BODY FROM GOING INTO LONG-TERM FIGHT OR FLIGHT.

LEARN TO SHIFT TO REST-AND-DIGEST MODE

To stop a migraine, it is critical to shift from fight-or-flight mode to rest-and-digest mode. The mind-body dance helps you be present and aware of the communication that must happen between the mind and body to feel well. When this balance occurs from your conscious effort, you automatically shift into the rest-and-digest state, which is critical for relieving migraine pain. Anytime you are in rest and digest, more resources are directed from the muscles back to the brain, and the brain eventually recovers and stops screaming in pain. This is the objective of the four steps of the *Stop, Drop, Roll, and Smile* method.

LOOK FOR UNDERLYING CAUSES OF YOUR SYMPTOMS

You may think chocolate, cheese, the weather, or something else is causing your migraines, but these triggers are hints that can reveal a much bigger picture. Triggers simply tip the scale in an already out-of-balance nervous system and possibly a poorly functioning liver. To heal the body from ever having another migraine, please see my book *The Migraine Protocol*. In that book, you will learn all you need to heal completely. Check my website at RealMigraineSolutions.com for current information on how to heal migraines and my next book, coming soon, which contains more information on healing migraines and my story.

WHERE WILL YOU GO FROM HERE?

Using the *Stop*, *Drop*, *Roll*, *and Smile* method to derail a migraine or headache is the first step toward understanding what causes migraines and realizing that you have the power to do something about them. With practice and healing, migraines are completely preventable. Understand that you can heal yourself of the underlying causes of migraines and look forward to a life free of this debilitating pain.

Healing takes your commitment and dedication. It won't happen overnight for most people, but you can heal quickly if you find the right way to get the resources to your central nervous system. It will be a process of getting well and feeling better and better as you spend more time in a state of rest and digest—with proper breathing, smiling, and less resistance.

You must find your own balance and determine what creates that balance for you. That can take some trial and error. The most important takeaway is that **you can be completely migraine-free.** You deserve to enjoy a pain-free, fulfilling life. If you feel that you already have that, you have accomplished the most important step and with practice, the healing will follow.

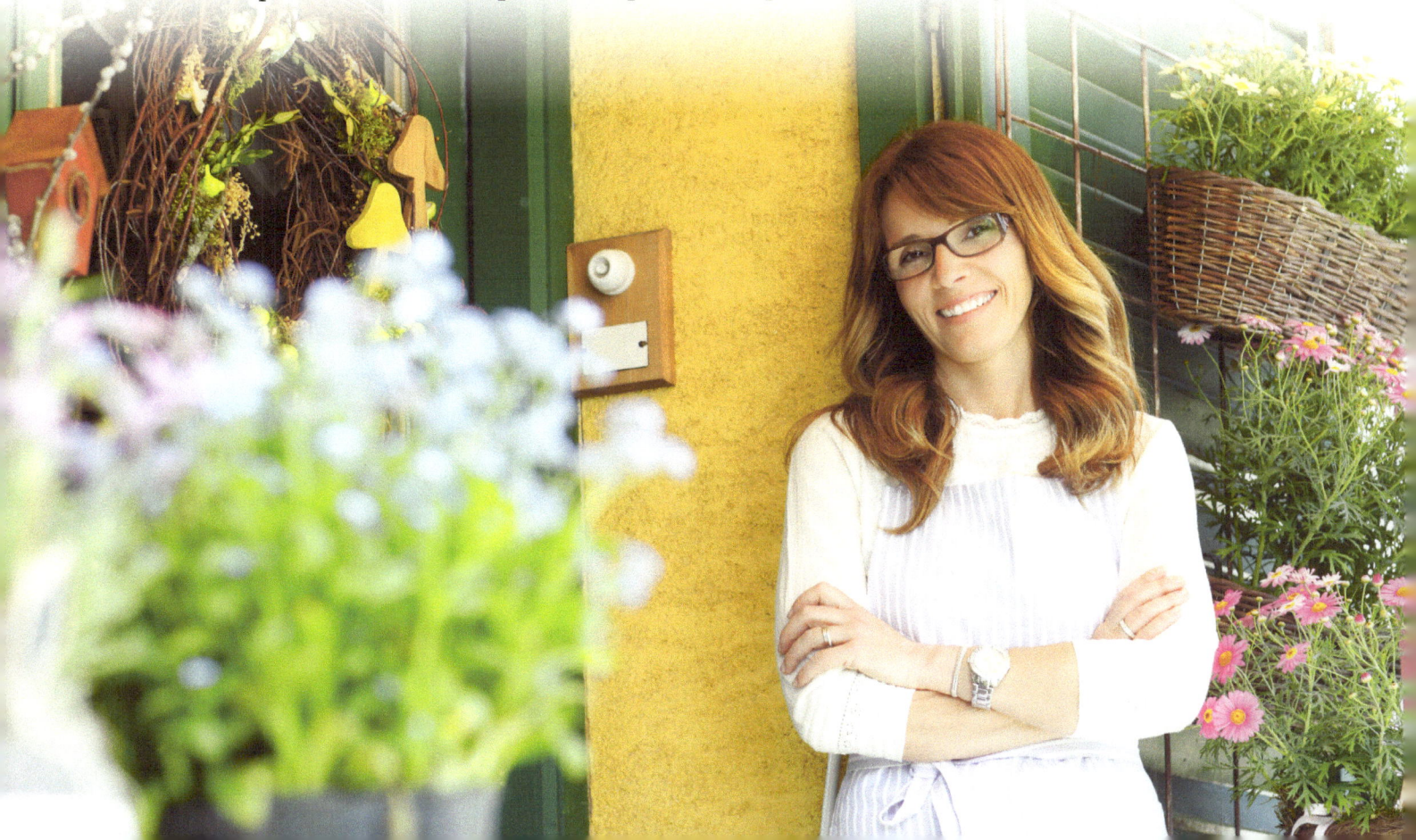

THE SIMPLE, EFFECTIVE STEPS
OUTLINED IN THIS MANUAL INCLUDE
GOOD BREATHING HABITS, GOOD
THOUGHTS, SMILING OFTEN,
AND OTHER POSITIVE PRACTICES
TO KEEP YOUR BODY IN
REST-AND-DIGEST MODE.

BONUS MATERIAL

COMMIT TO THE CURE

To get well and eliminate migraines from your life, commit to a new routine and be willing to make lifestyle choices to heal your body. The simple, effective steps outlined in this manual include good breathing habits, good thoughts, smiling often, and other positive practices to keep your body in rest-and-digest mode. Even if stress is not the main cause of your migraines, and they are caused by liver issues or thick blood or neck issues, your body can heal these ailments only when you are in a calm state of rest and digest. Getting well requires you to learn how to spend a lot of time with a calm nervous system.

Harness the Power of Words

In the process of healing, you may need to change your language to yourself and others. How you express yourself makes a huge difference.

Instead of telling others how bad your migraines are, teach your own brain something new by changing what you say. "I am doing better all of the time." "I feel great today." "I don't have migraines anymore." Say that before it is true, and eventually it will *be* true. Once I knew I was on the right path to my own healing, I used this to finally free myself from migraines.

The power of your words influences your health, mood, body, and reality—they give energy and meaning to what you experience. Your words can support your improving health, and the pain will diminish because of the actions you take and also the words you say. Commit to being well and then commit to it daily with your words and actions. Don't mention migraines because it gives energy to the pain instead of to your health. Your words are powerful and your body will respond to them.

WHEN YOU HAVE A MIGRAINE

When you have a full-blown migraine or headache, you have a big fire that is hard to control. Self-care is critical to releasing the pain as quickly as possible. Expand all steps of the Stop,

Drop, Roll, and Smile method. You must rest and relax the nervous system to stop the pain. Resting in a dark room is definitely helpful, but there is so much more you can do to assist your overtaxed, undernourished nervous system.

> Long periods of time at the computer, overthinking, hours of analyzing, or working without breaks can all "overheat" the brain from an excess of firing neurons. When the brain gets too hot, it burns through the resources very quickly, and like an overheated engine, it needs time and resources to cool off. It is unhealthy for the brain to get too hot, as brain cells are very sensitive to heat and can be damaged or die. Replenishing the resources and taking time to cool off the brain with sleep, rest, hydration, and breath are key to protecting the cells of the most important organ in your body.

Below are many ideas to help you shift the nervous system from fight or flight into rest and digest. Until you make this shift, you are using resources in a system that is out of fuel.

Here is an expanded list of things to do immediately when you have a migraine:

1. STOP to hydrate and relax—*Oranges, coconut water, watermelon, celery, minerals with glucose. Turmeric added to the foods you eat can also assist with hydration by providing easy-to-absorb vitamins and minerals.*

"Super" hydration includes water with natural glucose and minerals from juices or high water content fruits such as orange juice, coconut water, celery or celery juice, or watermelon. These liquids from nature contain high amounts of minerals with some glucose. Tap water doesn't necessarily hydrate cells. If your body is out of balance with low minerals, the water you are drinking may not enter the cells to hydrate them. Cells need the right mineral balance to allow for new water to move in and old water to exit the cell. Drinking fresh fruit juice or vegetable juice will provide minerals and water, which is what the cells need for thorough hydration. If juice is not accessible to you, add something such as Emergen-C to your water and of course, drink plain water if neither is available.

When hydrating, choose foods and drinks that hydrate and thin the blood. This is especially important if you have food triggers for your migraines. Blood-thinning foods are generally those that would wash down the sink with cold water. Blood-thickening foods generally need lots of hot water to wash down the sink, otherwise they will plug the drain (just like they can in the body).

Examples of blood-thinning foods are juice, fruit, vegetables, and soup. Blood thickening foods are butter, peanut butter, coconut oil, animal fat, and cheese. There are exceptions, such as alcohol that washes down the drain easily but also thickens the blood.

In general, blood-thinning foods are fruits and vegetables that are low in vitamin K (avoid leafy greens), and foods that are low in saturated and animal fats. High water content foods help in this regard, such as soups.

You can find a list of blood-thinning foods on my website at RealMigraineSolutions.com.

Be calm and reduce *all* stress—don't rush or allow daily pressure to get to you. Be grounded and fully present. See the relaxation techniques that follow.

2. DROP into belly breathing using the diaphragm—exhaling fully using long, slow exhales with a sigh. How to do this was covered well in Step 2.

Proper breathing may take practice. Spending hours a day sitting impedes deep breathing. Breathing deeply throughout the day often takes conscious effort. Eventually it becomes an automatic habit. Until it does become habit, be conscious of your breath throughout the day. Release a deep, relaxing sigh several times throughout the day. Anytime you notice that your breath has become shallow, spend a couple of minutes doing deep breathing with deep sighs of release. Set a timer to remind you to check your breathing. Getting well takes commitment. Until you inhale enough oxygen and exhale enough carbon dioxide, migraines and headaches are a threat.

You can find more information about deep breathing at RealMigraineSolutions.com and from my videos on YouTube.

3. ROLL—relax the muscles in the neck and spine. Learn what helps you to relax your muscles rapidly.

Prolonged sitting is one of the most common problems with neck issues, as it limits the entire spinal movement and the neck or low back may take the burden off of the other muscles. Proper neck alignment is critical for allowing nerve and blood flow to the head. Frequent stretching helps, as well as neck and back exercises. You may need to see a therapist for some added assistance.

4. SMILE and feel gratitude—even though it is hard to feel it when you are in pain. The physical act of smiling releases stress-counteracting hormones such as serotonin.

LEARN WHAT RELAXES YOU

Tension is like a rubber band that is wound up. It takes time for the band to unwind. You may need to take an hour to unwind and use several different techniques, depending on what is causing the tension. The value of finding time to unwind is priceless. Your brain must have downtime for the maintenance of the cells. It can only repair and keep the brain working properly with proper rest and relaxation. While you are using your brain, it cannot renew or heal itself.

Here are some possible ways to release tension and what to do when you feel a migraine coming on. If you are in a location where you can't do some of these steps, then do what you can do.

Stress-Relieving Activities

1. Take a warm bath and rub castor oil on sore muscles. Applying it in the tub will prevent the castor oil from staining your clothing, bedding, or furniture. Simply wash it off with soap before you get out of the tub and dry off. Castor oil has a magical effect that is not well understood. It relieves pain by increasing the flow of blood and lymph. (Note: If the body overheats, a migraine will get worse, so don't let the bath water be too hot. Take a bath in the early stages of a headache or migraine for a short duration. Getting overheated will cause blood to be directed to the organs to cool the body, so the brain gets less oxygen. A full-blown migraine can get worse as the blood is pulled away from the brain to cool off the body. Also, hydrate while you are in the tub.)

2. Rub White Flower oil (actually a blend of essential oils) on sore, tight muscles. This is the name of a product available on Amazon and at many health food stores. This formula has saved me from mountains of pain by increasing circulation to tired or tense muscles. It also promotes relaxed breathing. It is cheap and effective. Try it and help yourself recover quickly from tight muscles.

3. Rest relieves both muscles and nerves and allows more blood to flow to the brain.

4. Undulate the spine from the hips to the top of the head for several minutes, back and forth. This helps relax the entire spine. (If you are at work you may need to go into a bathroom stall so coworkers don't wonder what you are doing.) A link to my video demonstration of this exercise is listed in the Resources section.

5. Help your neck muscles to relax by doing gentle self-massage, resting your neck while sitting or lying down, doing gentle stretches and arm movements, and anything else that works to relax muscles and allow more blood to the head. Interestingly, tension

in the neck can actually begin in your feet, calves, and hamstrings. You may feel it as neck pain when in fact your entire body is tight. This can be caused by dehydration, as your fascia releases water to hydrate your organs when they are dehydrated and then can become tight and rigid as a result.

6. Belly breathe with eyes closed for 5-20 minutes minimum. Exhale fully to expel the buildup of carbon dioxide in lungs and blood. Allow the exhales to be longer than the inhales. This automatically relaxes the body. Focus on making your breath very slow. Picture a balloon in your lower abdomen and try to fill that balloon with air. Make the balloon slightly larger with each inhale, inflating the balloon. See the balloon completely deflate upon each exhalation. Did you push all of the air out of the balloon? Can you push out any more air? You could visualize something else instead of the balloon. Your breath could be the ocean waves, coming into shore on the inhale, water running up the beach as far as it can. On the exhale, the water trails out to the sea to blend into the smooth expansive liquid. Chose a picture of breath movement that works for you. Relax your shoulders and jaw a little more with each breath.

7. Professional massage, especially upper back, neck, and shoulders, helps relax the muscles so blood can flow better to the head.

8. Calming scents and music or anything relaxing works well also.

9. Being very present with your body, letting go of negative thoughts and worry, and relaxing your mind so you are in the moment and feeling your body is very powerful for the healing process. If you don't already know how to do this, it is a valuable process to learn.

10. Sexual release. If you can make love or even masturbate early on, before a migraine has developed, you can release some tension and move vital spinal fluid up the spine toward the head. A full-body orgasm is needed to move this energy and fluid the best.

Self-Care

11. Hydration increases blood flow to the brain. Water is the most valuable. Alcohol steals hydration from the body, as does coffee and caffeine-containing teas. Stick to juice and water and some herbal teas.

12. The underlying causes of migraines are beyond the scope of this manual, but if your migraines are triggered by certain foods, eat blood-thinning food like fruit and watery foods. Avoid saturated fats and vitamin K.

13. Take feverfew and hawthorn berry supplements to promote circulation. These work by supporting and healing the nervous system and vascular system. Be sure to buy high-quality supplements from a reputable source.

14. Avoid all pharmaceutical drugs, as much as you can, after consulting with your doctor. Prescription Sumatriptan is known to increase headaches. Hydrocodone may as well, over time, due to damage to the liver. The more time away from taking these harmful drugs, and any drugs, will help prevent future headaches. Sometimes the body may have to heal the damage to the vascular system from years of prescription drugs, which can take a while. During the time you are healing, you should be able to manage headache pain with the remedies listed in this manual.

15. Take calcium and magnesium supplements. When your body is in fight-or-flight mode and during a migraine, magnesium and calcium are released from your body into the urine. These electrolytes relax the muscles, which the body doesn't want during fight or flight. You may be deficient in these minerals, so include them along with hydration. As your nervous system relaxes, oxygen increases and pain begins to subside. If you tense up in response to the pain, this can slow down or stop the recovery. Breathe deeply to continue the healing. Magnesium and calcium can help your body stay calm, allow muscles to relax, and let the body recover from the effects of the near-migraine. My favorite product is NOW Colloidal Liquid Minerals, taken in juice or water. It is easy to take and is absorbed immediately. See the Resources section for more information.

IF YOU WANT TO REDUCE OR ELIMINATE YOUR MIGRAINE HEADACHES: LONG-TERM HEALING

The following information is covered in more depth in *The Migraine Protocol,* which includes a simple test to help you determine the underlying causes of your migraines plus my protocols for healing your body from the identified causes. The more you understand about your body's response to stress and how it heals itself, the better you are able to help your body heal and then stay healthy.

Fight-or-Flight Mode Can Be Triggered by More Than Stress

Some people believe visualization, meditation, relaxation, happy thoughts, belly breathing, extra sleep, and calming music will always work and can eventually keep you out of a sympathetic (fight-or-flight) state. However, threats to your health such as a pinched vertebral nerve and/or artery, damaged TMJ joint, overtaxed liver, or damaged vascular system can cause your body to go into fight or flight because the brain perceives a threat. You may be completely unaware of this. I have mentioned this before but it's worth repeating—deliberate relaxation is a necessary part of fighting migraines.

When you do not have enough circulation to the brain, it is difficult to tell the brain all is well. When this happens, you know your body needs healing. Deep, slow exhalations are the most powerful way to calm the body and allow the healing to begin.

YOUR BODY CANNOT HEAL OR MAKE NEW CELLS UNLESS IT IS *RELAXED.*

Once your migraine is gone, it is time to figure out what the brain is perceiving as a threat and fix the underlying issue.

Healing Takes Time

If your migraines are caused by something other than stress, your body must heal before you have consistent and adequate blood flow to the brain. It may take some time to retrain your brain not to react to nonthreatening nerve impulses. Regardless of the cause, all healing occurs during relaxation.

While you retrain, you may still have migraines or headaches. Your body's path to healing may be unique to you. Whatever your healing journey turns out to be, if you follow the practices here, you will observe your headaches getting better, less painful, and less frequent and with a shorter duration.

While you are healing, be very conscious and aware of blood flow to the brain and keep it flowing by maintaining rest-and-digest mode as much as possible. Frequently move and stretch if you work at a desk, be gentle to your neck to avoid strain, and eat a good diet that is low in saturated or processed trans fats.

The headaches you may get while you heal have the same triggers and causes as your migraines. If you are down to less severe and less frequent headaches, then your body is already healing, and your vascular system is better able to circulate blood to the brain than it could before. If you have spinal alignment issues, then less pain may mean you are keeping your spine in better alignment. Soon you will be both headache- and migraine-free.

Healing Takes Commitment to the Changes

If you want to be completely well, you must commit to making this happen and making the changes needed. You must break a pattern. If you do, you will get well. All physical illness is caused by the same thing, to some degree, which is lack of oxygen from poor breathing and therefore low electrical conductivity. Every breath you take communicates signals to your nervous system regarding what to do with the resources available.

Migraines are a disease in the body . . . a body lacking ease (that is, time in rest-and-digest mode) and oxygen, which causes the nervous system to use up resources fast. When it comes to creating ease in the body, breathing properly with deep exhalation is the key, along with the practices listed here. Soon you will be back in balance and living life without migraines.

STOP
DROP
ROLL
SMILE

RESOURCES

Below are some resources that may support you on this healing journey.

Supplements

- Colloidal Minerals such as NOW brand, available in health nutrition centers and online, including Amazon. https://smile.amazon.com/NOW-Colloidal-Minerals-Liquid-32-Ounce/dp/B0013OXCU2/ref=sr_1_3?crid=33UL1JWSJUIKV&keywords=now+colloidal+minerals+liquid%2C32-ounce&qid=1558018315&s=hpc&sprefix=now+colloidal+%2Chpc%2C236&sr=1-3

Muscle Relaxing Creams and Oils

- White Flower Essential Oils. This link is for three bottles, which I always buy because I use this a lot, but you can also buy one bottle at a time on Amazon or your local health food store. https://smile.amazon.com/White-Flower-Balm-Oil-20ml/dp/B01CTFRA74/ref=sr_1_3?crid=2WNG2YL0HJGH&keywords=white+flower+essential+oil&qid=1558017161&s=hpc&sprefix=white+flower+esse%2Chpc%2C194&sr=1-3

- Oil-Free Arnica Liniment with ginger. This has a mild scent and works well also. https://smile.amazon.com/SUPER-SALVE-Arnica-Liniment-FZ/dp/B014Q32G1W/ref=smi_www_rco2_go_smi_g3905707922?_encoding=UTF8&%2AVersion%2A=1&%2Aentries%2A=0&ie=UTF8

- Castor Oil

Books

- *The Migraine Protocol* by Diana Anderson (Aloha Publishing, 2019)
- Coming soon: my new book on the five causes of migraines and how to heal them. See RealMigraineSolutions.com for more information.

Video/Audio

- YouTube Channel: https://www.youtube.com/channel/UCXf0BJQ2cIV8jFNLG0VORpg
- *Coming soon:* my soon-to-be-released video course can be accessed from RealMigraineSolutions.com
- Video on how to undulate the spine: https://www.youtube.com/watch?v=3tJzmK8MO8g&feature=youtu.be

ENDNOTES

1. Https://migraineresearchfoundation.org/about-migraine/migraine-facts/

2. Https://www.ncbi.nlm.nih.gov/pmc/articles/PMC3078506/

3. Https://www.ncbi.nlm.nih.gov/books/NBK22436/

4. Https://www.ncbi.nlm.nih.gov/books/NBK493232/

5. Https://articles.mercola.com/sites/articles/archive/2018/09/01/what-is-fascia.aspx

I APPRECIATE ALL THE
WONDERFUL PEOPLE IN MY
LIFE WHO HAVE CROSSED MY
PATH OR SUPPORTED ME.

ACKNOWLEDGMENTS

I would like to thank my mother, Tina Montee, for always being the first person to read and edit my books and fix all the glaring typos so I can feel confident enough to let others read a better version. She is a far better writer than I and everything about her life inspires me to live more fully and be more like her. I would like to thank my aunt Carla Siebel for always being the second person to read my books and find many ways I could improve them. Together they have lovingly and politely read many early drafts of my several works.

I am grateful for my dear sister, Jina Nelson, for her confidence in me, as well as her genuine support and encouragement. My three daughters always offer me their love and confidence. Their bright, beautiful spirits give me all of the motivation I need. Thank you my sweet daughters, Rebecca Kent, Christina Bartschi, and Shari DeVaard. I do nothing in this world without keeping you in mind!

With very few words, my father, Ken Montee, believes in me and wants nothing more than for his two daughters to receive what we desire. Thank you, Dad.

Thank you to my dear friends. Julie Lynn, for her confidence and support and for sharing how she healed herself from migraines with willpower and belief. She is a strong, incredible woman. Thanks to Narda Pitkethly for believing in me, giving me advice, and being a support. Narda's personal accomplishments show me that one person can make a tremendous difference in the world. I have many other amazing friends who have inspired me along the way: Jody Stanislaw, Julie Johnson, Kristen Schneck, Lynnette Jones, Ashiauna Louderbough, and Ann Peach.

I wish to thank several doctors for their contribution to my long-term health. My dear Dr. Michael Moriarty, who became my friend after putting me back together as my chiropractor for 35 years, following four separate car accidents. He started me on the path to understanding healing the body and good health practices. Dr. Steve Politis, who did minute adjustments in my neck to free up more blood traveling to my brain. I am forever grateful for his expertise and excellent training. He also reminded me to belly breathe when I had forgotten. Dr. Bart Goldman, who read my early draft of the full book and gave me his expert opinion and blessing. Bart was a great resource from the medical perspective.

Then I come to my blessed publishing team. I greatly appreciate Maryanna Young for taking an interest in my project and publishing the first products, such as this one. Maryanna is a visionary and expert in her industry. Of course, I could not have created a concise, logical structure without my fabulous editor, Jennifer Regner. She is brilliant at what she does.

I appreciate all the wonderful people in my life who have crossed my path or supported me. There are too many to name. Thankfully we don't travel this world alone. This material would not be available without the energy of many other beings, including all of those with migraines who allowed me to share this information to help them on their journey. I appreciate *all* the individuals who helped this work become available.

ABOUT THE AUTHOR

Diana Anderson lived with migraine headaches for her entire adult life, until the prescribed medications no longer relieved her pain. She also realized her headaches had been increasing in severity and frequency and she had more triggers than ever before—including being at higher altitudes and wearing a hat. She researched alternatives and sought out practitioners to help her regain her health. Over the course of almost three years, her learning journey brought her to a new understanding that migraine headaches were an indicator that something in the body needed healing. After healing herself, her intimate knowledge of migraine pain motivated her to write her knowledge down so she could share it and help others.

Diana is not content to lie still and watch the world happen around her. She enjoys experiencing life to the fullest and creating powerful memories. When migraines took the joy of life from her, she was absolutely determined to get her spark back.

Now that she has her spark back, she enjoys traveling the world, hiking, biking, floating the rivers, and spending time in the solitude of nature. When she is not in her flower garden, she is with friends or family, writing at her computer, or exploring this glorious planet. When given the opportunity, she also teaches at retreats, workshops, and courses about the tools she has found useful to enjoy a healthy, fulfilled life.

Her five grandkids call her Nana and they ride on her back, chase her around at the zoo, and help her tend to the garden. She is thankful for so many of life's unlimited wonders and the inspiring people around her. However, her greatest joys come from her family, especially her three brilliant daughters, her delightful, energetic grandkids, and her sons-in-law. She lives in Idaho, surrounded by the outdoors she loves to explore.

Diana is a prolific author. If you want to connect with her other products, see the list below. She has written two novels as well as three books for women on improving intimate pleasure with a partner. She has a course for men and a course for women on how to improve the connection in the bedroom as well as the pleasure and fun.

If you would like to contact Diana about a speaking or teaching engagement on the topic of migraines, health, or pleasure, visit RealMigraineSolutions.com

PLEASE SHARE THIS
INFORMATION WITH ANYONE
YOU KNOW WHO SUFFERS FROM
HEADACHES OR MIGRAINES.

CONNECT WITH ME

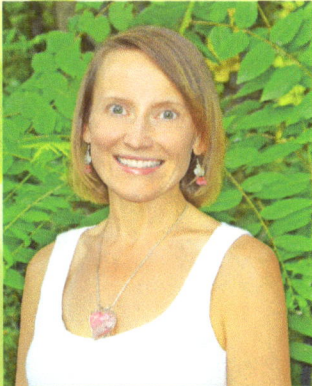

If this book helped you, I would love to hear from you. Connect with me on my Facebook group, on my Facebook page, on LinkedIn, or contact me through my website at RealMigraineSolutions.com.

Please share this information with anyone you know who suffers from headaches or migraines. Let others know how it helped you by posting a review on Amazon or Goodreads or by spreading the word on social media.

My hope is to reach as many people as possible with these simple steps toward making their lives better and less painful.

Be well. I hope your life is full of joy.

Diana Anderson

RealMigraineSolutions.com

Facebook group: Facebook.com/group/realmigrainesolutions/

Facebook: Facebook.com/dianamonteeanderson

LinkedIn: Diana Anderson, Real Estate Investment Specialist at KW Commercial in Boise, Idaho (https://www.linkedin.com/in/Diana-Anderson-96b07219/)

REALMIGRAINESOLUTIONS.COM

www.ingramcontent.com/pod-product-compliance
Lightning Source LLC
Chambersburg PA
CBHW060820270326
41930CB00003B/103